The
FLEX
Diet

JAMES BECKERMAN, M.D.

A TOUCHSTONE BOOK
Published by Simon & Schuster
New York   London   Toronto   Sydney

Touchstone
A Division of Simon & Schuster, Inc.
1230 Avenue of the Americas
New York, NY 10020

Designed by Renata Di Biase

Manufactured in the United States of America

ISBN 978-1-4391-5569-1

To Stacie, Jack, and Henry

Contents

INTRODUCTION

Doctors are problem solvers. Solving problems is what we do.

I never really set out to write a diet book. But things don't always happen the way you thought they would. This book was written because I started looking for some answers that I could use to help my patients—one patient in particular—with a common problem. Without a working solution.

Let me tell you a little bit about me to put things into perspective. I am a cardiologist—a heart specialist—working out of a large community teaching hospital tucked away in Portland, Oregon. I see patients—people like you—every single day. College students and pensioners, white- and blue-collar workers, single parents, boomers, cuspers, and increasingly Gen Xers. I meet them when they are in the office and in the ICU, on the examination table, off a helicopter, and sometimes on a ventilator.

A lot of what I do occurs after their wake-up call—a heart attack, a diagnosis of congestive heart failure, or the rapid palpitations of atrial fibrillation. There is a lot of excitement in *being there* during that moment to help someone make it to the next graduation, christening, or family vacation. But despite all the drama, I have always felt that the greatest impact occurs *outside* the fluorescence of the cardiac catheterization lab and away from the rhythms of intravenous medications and ventilators. It happens in the outpatient setting, when people are feeling good and optimistic and confident, when they have time to ask and listen, and when I have the opportunity to share some opinions, write prescriptions, and occasionally offer some solutions.

This book is dedicated to my patients.

My patients are real people. They don't give testimony on infomercials—they are the ones watching them. They don't have cooks or coaches. They work, they chase after their kids, and they need every bit of sleep they can get. They eat French fries. Some smoke. They make difficult choices and sometimes make mistakes. *They are looking for solutions.* And sometimes they give me the privilege of listening to their questions and helping them understand their problems.

What do you ask *your* doctor?

In any patient-doctor encounter, each person has goals. Your doctor might focus on your abnormal liver function tests, whether or not you are up to date on your colonoscopy, making sure he isn't late for the next patient, or . . . his afternoon tee time. But what are *your* goals? If you don't know, you are definitely at a disadvantage.

When we go to the doctor, we are brought by symptoms, referred by fear, and often intimidated by rising co-pays and, subsequently, blood pressure. But I am amazed when I ask someone who has come to see me, "So, what brings you here today?" only to be faced with an uncertain stare or a puzzled look. People seem genuinely surprised at the question sometimes, and often do not have an answer. But I keep pressing them on it, and am often surprised by what I hear.

CAN YOU HELP ME LOSE WEIGHT?

The first time I was asked this, I was honestly taken aback. I am a cardiologist, not a miracle worker! I thought my job was to mend broken hearts, get people through surgery, and make them dizzy with blood pressure medication and resentful toward me for taking away their bacon cheeseburgers. I didn't get into this to solve people's weight concerns. I would rather leave that for someone else with more time, more patience, and maybe even his own television show.

But I slowly began to realize something.

Sure, people want to be healthy. No one wants to be hospitalized with a heart attack or watch a loved one undergo open-heart surgery for a problem that might have been prevented. No one wants high blood pressure or diabetes. No one wants to take medicines. No one wants to be tired all day or feel lousy performing simple tasks.

But it's hard to feel your blood pressure.

It's hard to see your cholesterol or blood sugar.

However, there is a cardiac risk factor that stares you in the face each and every time you go to brush your teeth, put on (or take off) some clothes, or ask someone out on a date (or wait to be asked out). Your weight.

Your weight is a barometer of your health, including your heart health. People care deeply about their weight, and for lots of different reasons. And heart health usually is not one of them. That's okay with me, though. It doesn't matter if our motivations are different, just as long as our *solution* is the same. I don't mind getting to your heart through your stomach, as the saying goes. Just so long as I get there.

FROM "ON LOCATION" TO ONLINE

After a few years of exploring these issues and challenges in my cardiology clinic, I felt increasingly stumped by what appeared to be a universal concern. People want to have a good quality of life, but making good choices sometimes seems to make life harder and less satisfying. When you stare down at your belly while standing on the scale, losing the excess weight can seem like an impossible task. This goes for pretty much everyone. It is not just about heart disease; it is about feeling confident when you walk into a club, socialize with friends, or return to work after maternity leave. It is about feeling comfortable in your own skin, and your own clothes. It is about doing things safely and for the long term.

It is about time . . . isn't it?

I started talking with more patients, and more people generally, about their concerns. I visited Rotary clubs and community forums and spoke to folks about heart disease prevention and making better choices. I engaged friends and strangers on blogs, boards, Facebook, and Twitter. I even started posting my own insights (and occasional rants) on the Web at www.jamesbeckerman.com—come by and visit sometime.

Recognizing that this universal problem extended far beyond my little corner of the Pacific Northwest, I decided to take it on the road— the Internet highway, to be more specific—and interact with patients outside the physical scope of my clinical practice. I became the Heart Expert at www.WebMD.com and the Weight Loss / Healthy Living Expert at www.MedHelp.org, where you can find me every day answering questions about heart disease, weight loss, and living a healthy life. With millions of unique visitors each month, these websites provide a trustworthy resource for medical information and news. I have been impressed by the insights provided by the members of the community message boards, where readers create their own content and share their experiences. And I am constantly amazed by the thoughtfulness of the posts I get to read and respond to.

Add to this a growing cardiology practice that has continued to evolve with a heavy emphasis on cardiac risk factor modification, lifestyle choices, and healthy eating. Things got busy. Just ask my wife and toddlers. But, like you, I strive for balance, and I thought I had it figured out. And then I met Mr. S. and nothing was the same after that.

A SINGLE PATIENT, A SINGLE SOLUTION

Let me tell you about Mr. S. You probably know a lot of guys like him. Or maybe he's your brother, coworker, or spouse. He is in his forties. He travels a lot for work but lives for his kids. He plays guitar. He wants to make it to the gym more often.

And that's where he was when his heart stopped. He was getting ready to climb on the elliptical trainer and had a cardiac arrest before he pressed "Start."

Fortunately, there were lots of people around to help him. Unfortunately, his son was one of them. Bystanders provided CPR until emergency medical personnel arrived. Mr. S. was found to be in ventricular fibrillation, a frequently lethal cardiac rhythm in which the heart is unable to supply the brain with blood. Or oxygen.

Mr. S. was shocked into normal rhythm, and he was brought by ambulance into the emergency department, where I met him one Tuesday afternoon. His electrocardiogram showed that he was having a heart attack, and he was rushed to the cardiac catheterization laboratory, where the small coronary artery supplying the front of his heart with blood was found to be closed. It was opened without difficulty, and a small metal stent was inserted to keep the blood vessel open so that his damaged heart muscle could receive oxygen. However, his blood pressure failed to stabilize; he needed a breathing tube and a slew of medications just to stay alive.

He had trouble waking up. Family and friends visited, and we were all discouraged, despite our attempts at hope. Too much time without a heartbeat. Not enough oxygen. It really was not looking like a happy ending to his story.

But then it happened. Small changes led to bigger ones. His breathing status somehow improved. He came off the ventilator. After days of confusion and delirium, Mr. S. asked for his guitar, and we all could breathe again. By the time he was discharged from the hospital, I was thrilled to see him leave on his own terms, and on his own two feet, even though he was slow to speak and he shuffled when he walked.

I didn't think much about Mr. S. until a month later. In the meantime, there were lots of heart attacks. Lots of heart catheterizations. And occasionally some bad outcomes. So I was pretty excited to see him on my clinic schedule for a follow-up visit.

It was remarkable. If you had never seen this guy before, you would not have guessed how close to death he had been just a few weeks earlier. He appeared strong and confident, and he realized how lucky he was. After we'd gone over his medications and made plans for our next appointment, he paused before putting on his coat.

"But can you help me get rid of this?" With a sheepish grin, he pointed to his gut and laughed. Right then, it hit me. Here was this guy, who some would argue was really the luckiest guy in the world. He was gone and then he came back, had a touch-and-go hospitalization, and would have been fortunate to even be able to remember his own name. But now, after cutting-edge technology had restored his heart function and helped bring his mind back to reality, here we were discussing his waistline as if he were a college student lamenting the "freshman fifteen." After this whole ordeal, it came back to the belly. Sure, he had other risk factors for future heart problems, but his weight was *his* greatest concern. And he was now ready to do something about it. He was motivated to make a change. I decided then and there: I have to do something to help Mr. S. and others like him. And *unlike* him.

COMMON PROBLEM, MANY SOLUTIONS

One thing I've learned from taking care of loggers and executives, grandmothers and kids just out of high school is that you can't treat everyone the same way, even if they have the same problem. A truck driver might have a different perspective on his blood pressure medication regimen ("No water pill, please") than a software engineer. A single mom with three kids will see the world differently from a retiree trying to improve his or her quality of life above all else. We recognize this diversity every day in health care, and we change our approaches and sometimes our actual therapies to achieve the same results. If heart medications and invasive procedures can be tailored to individuals, then it seems to me that healthy lifestyle choices can be too.

In a culture of evolving individuality—from our shoes to our smartphones—we each expect to experience the world in our own unique way, even if a common approach is cheaper or more readily available. This is in direct contrast to previous generations, when there were fewer choices and people had fewer expectations. Today, we are searching for more possibilities, and we want an individualized, personalized experience in everything we do.

Although I originally set out to create a solution for weight loss and a healthy lifestyle that could work for Mr. S. and other patients in my clinic, I soon recognized that a truly innovative solution would have to work for anyone and everyone, whether you are younger or older, male or female, active or sedentary, vegan or carnivore, an experienced dieter or just interested in trying something new. In order to make it universal, I had to make it personalized. The Flex Diet may have been created for Mr. S., but it was written for everyone else. Including you.

SINGLE POUND, SINGLE STEP

We are used to thinking about our destination before we plan our route. Our goals exist before we figure out how to reach them. And we sometimes dream about where we want to be without paying attention to where we are right now.

So if losing weight is your objective, how you go about it may not seem important to you. But setting your goal is really your challenge. Because you *do* have to figure out how to get to it.

How do you lose ten, twenty, or even fifty pounds? What can you eat? How much exercise do you really have to do? The difficulty of figuring it all out seems insurmountable. The mountain always does when you are sitting at the bottom, staring at the summit. But if you take a moment and look at the path, you can find short goals along the way to keep you interested. To keep you engaged. To keep you inspired. To keep you going.

As you open this book, and turn these first pages, you are in a sense beginning a journey. It may be a journey that you have begun many times before. And you do not need to be acquainted with ancient Chinese proverbs to know that this journey, like so many others, begins with a single step.

With a single pound.

Weight loss *is* the goal. It is a number. It is a dress size. It is a deadline.

But contrary to what some weight-loss programs might suggest, you cannot live your life day to day with only the big picture in mind. It is too hard to stay on the path. It becomes too easy to make a misstep and feel that you have to start over again.

The truth is, we live our lives without having an overarching plan, but instead by being nimble and flexible. We make a seemingly infinite number of small choices, many of which we don't even recognize. And they take us, slowly or quickly, closer to or farther away from where we genuinely want to be. Even though we want to fulfill whatever promise we make to ourselves, our *strategy* will be reaching our goal *step by step*, rather than trying to leap toward it in a single bound, only to realize in midair that we can't actually fly.

Losing weight begins with *a single pound*.

Eat. Drink. Exercise. Act. *Live*. Once you understand the two hundred different weight-loss Solutions presented in the chapters that follow, you can combine them to reach your own personal goals. Be flexible. Remember, one pound at a time. To keep you going. Toward where you want to be.

It's the Flex Diet. It bends so *you* won't break.

1

START WITH A SINGLE POUND

It is not the mountain we conquer, but ourselves.

— Sir Edmund Hillary

You picked up this book for a reason.

You are tired of the same old approach.

You have had enough of advertisements, pop-up ads, and celebrity endorsements. Your bookshelf is full of laminated cards, cookbooks, systems, how-tos, and self-helps. Your kitchen feels sugar-free, fat-free, and taste-free. You are distracted and maybe even disheartened, but *still* are planning to try again next Monday. And your pants don't fit right.

You picked up this book because it's time for a solution.

You might be browsing in the bookstore or on the Internet. You may have heard about this book from a friend. You may even be one of my patients. It doesn't matter how you got here, as long as you get where you want to be.

You could be anyone. A bridesmaid-to-be or a recent college graduate dreading that first reunion. A new mom who wants to get off the baby weight. An executive on the road with a steady diet of steak and Scotch. A retiree who wants to spend more time out of the house. Or maybe you have just had a heart attack and are trying to make things right.

Welcome to the Flex Diet, a fresh approach to the same old problem. No calorie counting. No scales. No points. The Flex Diet operates on a simple principle that you can apply throughout your life: small changes yield big results. But they have to work for *you*. For the next eight weeks, you will choose among two hundred different Solutions to lose twenty pounds.

You already know that weight loss is not easy. No matter how you approach it, a diet requires you to change your life. That's just being honest. But the Flex Diet is the first integrated weight loss program that lets *you* decide how you are going to do it.

PEOPLE ARE NOT PARADIGMS

People are by nature impatient. And there are a lot of diet books in recycling bins and landfills that will attest to that. With bookshelves and websites offering unlimited advice, there is too much noise, but there are not enough clear calls to action. Writers, gurus, and even doctors are so busy trying to sell us on the next big thing that they miss an opportunity to *teach* us skills that we can individually apply to our lives.

We end up treating weight loss like a game show instead of a path to wellness. Diets are things to "start" and to "be on," and all the rewards, gold stars, and immunity challenges excite us into feeling as if we have already succeeded even if we never lose a single pound. This is great entertainment, but the problem is, once you tire of the gimmick, there has to be something there to keep you going.

Eating bacon-wrapped cheese-stuffed sausage rolls is not one of those things.

The reason it is so hard to maintain diets is that you feel you are making too much of a departure from the way you normally live your life in order to participate in a foreign ritual or system—and that is exactly why it is so easy to quit. And if you were to make one mistake, eat one wrong thing, or inhale too deeply in the bakery section, you might ruin this artificial world that has been created for you. Once you return to food "reality," you remember that you like it. And the minute you put away the chart, lose the portion scale, or hide the flour substitute, you are back to raiding the pantry for Good N Plenty candies and then staring blankly in the mirror before deciding once again to start all over on Monday. But it's not Monday that you should be worried about. It's next Thursday, or that long tailgating weekend at the University of Desperation.

Don't get me wrong. There are lots of great diet books out there that have helped people lose millions of pounds. But you need to know what you are getting yourself into. You can identify the fads by their hook, whether it be consuming fewer [insert food here], more [insert food here], or eating [more/less] frequently in [larger/smaller] portions until you go [insane/crazy]. Paradigm shifts work well when it comes to thinking about the shape of the Earth or how giraffes got such long necks, but not when it comes to strict rules about carbohydrates, "superfoods," or protein shakes that belong in a science experiment rather than in your kitchen—or stomach.

People are not paradigms that can be shifted. The Flex Diet encourages you to be an individual, and it celebrates that fact by asking *you* to make the personal choices that will get you where you want to be—thinner, healthier, and more energetic. Individualized choices are more sustainable and more empowering than a rigid set of rules that can't be followed by everyone. You can wrap your mind around the choices you make, and if some of them do not ultimately agree with your lifestyle, you can pass on them but still maintain a benefit from the eight-week program.

It's time to introduce the Solutions. When I first started thinking about how to communicate the building blocks of a healthy lifestyle to my own patients, I was overwhelmed by how to approach it the right way. How can you really look someone in the eye and explain *everything* that needs to be done to lose a hundred pounds? It's more than daunting. But let's change the focus away from the number and toward the program's individual elements. Anyone can lose a single pound. And this program will teach you how to do just that. In two hundred different ways.

Solutions range from the obvious to the intriguing, from common sense to cutting-edge science, with just the right amount of "outside the box" thinking to make it fun. Hundreds of scientific studies have been dissected and distilled so that you will read only about what works and why. And the best part is that if a particular Solution is not for you, you can keep reading until you find others that fit your lifestyle and your goals. That's where the Flex comes into play. So let's get started. Your Solutions are organized into three phases of an eight-week journey: Today, Every Day, and *Your* Way.

FLEX

Every time you see the **FLEX** symbol throughout this book, you have another opportunity to make this program your own. The Flex Solutions are yours to choose from—several will be presented, and you only need to try one to get the benefit. And if you decide not to stick with it, just substitute another Flex Solution. I won't tell anyone.

TODAY

Weeks One and Two: Five Pounds

In medical practice there is a concept called the teachable moment. Such moments occur at key points in the interaction between patients and the health care system, and they offer our best opportunities to help people make healthy choices. For example, there is a teachable moment when people are discharged from the hospital, since they are motivated to get better and are thinking about their health with fewer distractions. This becomes the best time to get someone to stop smoking or start cholesterol medication. Other teachable moments occur in the doctor's office or even over the telephone. The idea is that people are most likely to make changes in their lives during those moments when they are focused on their goals.

Welcome to your teachable moment.

Because *today* is when you are most likely to start making changes. So, in the Today chapter, you will find easy-to-incorporate Solutions that will help you start losing weight right now. If you follow all these Solutions, expect to lose five pounds in the next two weeks. Five pounds that shouldn't come back. The Today Solutions are your blueprint to start building a new you.

EVERY DAY

Weeks Three, Four, and Five: Ten Pounds

Every Day Solutions are the cornerstones of wellness, prevention, and serious weight loss. They are intended for everyone, and they should be compatible with your lifestyle. These scientifically proven Solutions will help you lose ten more pounds in just three weeks. Nearly one hundred different opportunities are blended together into one comprehensive three-week plan that works for everyone. Every day.

The Solutions are organized into the five "senses" of wellness: Eating, Drinking, Exercise, Activity, and Lifestyle. Solutions at the beginning of each section are meant for everyone, while the Flex Solutions presented later in the section are your opportunity to personalize your program. Choose at least one Flex Solution from each section to incorporate into your Every Day.

YOUR WAY

Weeks Six, Seven, Eight, and Beyond: How Much Weight Do *You* Want to Lose?

This is where it really starts to get interesting. After two weeks concentrating on the Today Solutions and three more weeks working through the Every Day Solutions, you are looking and feeling great. You might be happy to stop right here. But if you want to take things up a notch and also have some fun, let's get personal. Or at least get *personalized*. Spend three weeks on a personal reboot with nearly one hundred more Solutions at your disposal. Choose ten more ways to Eat, Drink, Exercise, Act, and Live *your* way toward at least five more pounds of weight loss, a single pound at a time. And if a Solution isn't working out for you, just Flex it for another. The Flex Diet bends so *you* won't break. Either way, you win, and you will succeed.

So what do *you* have to lose? Start by losing the lectures. Lose the exchanges. And lose the points. Hold on to your Solutions and turn the page to a healthier life and a slimmer waistline. Start losing weight *your* way.

Because you picked up this book for a reason.

Now find your Solution.

Because Today is Monday.

2.

TODAY

Apparently there is nothing that cannot happen today.

— MARK TWAIN

The goal of Today is to get you started with Solutions you can use right now. You may have even skipped to this chapter just to cut to the chase—I don't blame you at all. This section lays out the Solutions that you should start following for the next two weeks so that you can start seeing results—*today*. Each Solution is easy to do, and makes sense. If you like, you can read through the expanded discussion of each Solution if you want a deeper understanding of the research and reasoning behind it. But not everyone wants a science lesson. It is up to you how much you want to get into it.

These Solutions emphasize the concept of mindfulness. We are constantly making hundreds of lifestyle choices throughout the day—from choosing stairs over the elevator to what kind of milk we put in our coffee. And research suggests that when we are more engaged in the process of making choices—if we are consciously aware that those choices exist—we tend to make better decisions. We get into trouble when we are distracted or become forgetful. The trick is to remain plugged in without concentrating on the diet twenty-four hours a day.

The only thing harder than going on a diet is listening to someone *else* go on a diet. Hearing about points, exchanges, and calories burned on the treadmill is way too much information. So our goal is to avoid becoming similarly obsessed, and instead incorporate mindfulness into the program in more subtle ways. Because mindfulness leads to compliance. And compliance is what keeps us making good decisions in two weeks, two months, and beyond. Mindfulness is why the Today Solutions are built for success.

The whole idea behind the Today Solutions is that they are things that you can literally start doing once you read the list that follows. The key is to start *today*. It doesn't matter what day of the week you are reading this. It doesn't matter if you have a date tonight. It doesn't matter if you are going to a wedding this weekend. Start today and you will lose five pounds—and probably even more—by the end of two weeks.

Ready to find *your* Solution?

THE TODAY SOLUTIONS

1. Commit yourself by taking a photo.
2. Join a support group.
3. Use automated reminders.
4. Tatango!
5. Get a commitment from your significant other.
6. Find a weight-loss buddy.
7. Follow people who inspire you on Twitter.
8. Become someone's coach.
9. Blog.
10. Call your doctor.
11. Weigh yourself daily.
12. Warm up.
13. Keep a food diary.
14. Drink six glasses of water a day.
15. Take a multivitamin.
16. Get your calcium.
17. Consider taking fish oil.
18. Look into probiotics.
19. Try taking whey protein after exercise.

20. Wear a pedometer.
21. Don't use exercise as a punishment.
22. Almonds.
23. Apples.
24. Grapes.
25. Greek yogurt.
26. Flaxseeds.
27. Pine nuts.
28. Enjoy 100-calorie snacks.
29. Don't overdose on energy bars.
30. Close the kitchen after dinner.
31. Sleep at least seven hours a night.

Solution #1

Commit Yourself by Taking a Photo

Draw a line in the sand today, and start by understanding what you want to accomplish. We are so goal-oriented that we do not pay enough attention to where we are right now. Take a photo, and use it as a starting point.

Documenting your weight-loss journey keeps you mindful and rewards your progress. Because when push comes to shove and that cinnamon roll seems like a pretty good bedtime snack, there is nothing like a glossy eight-by-ten to get you motivated. Having a handy photo of yourself at a less desirable weight helps you remember your goals, especially during those difficult moments.

Take a photo of yourself today. You can use your cell phone or digital camera, and if you really want to make an impact, print it out. You do not need to wear a bathing suit or an unflattering outfit; just keep it real and keep it away from Photoshop. Put it in your bathroom or on your refrigerator; use it as your desktop background or on your phone. And then at thirty, sixty, and ninety days, take another photo in the same setting—no tanning or professional lighting allowed to augment reality. There won't be a need. Because the picture will say a thousand words.

Don't Do It Alone!

Anyone who has been around the diet block once or twice knows that it can be lonely at the salad bar. It's easy to feel isolated when you make the decision to start living your life differently. One of your challenges right now is that your girlfriends would rather go out for margaritas than to a yoga class, and your kids or spouse won't even touch a salad. Research shows that having support is key in being successful with a diet. And the exciting thing about going on a diet *today* is that you have more choices than ever in how to avoid going at it alone. Flex one of the following eight Solutions to get other people involved. Chances are, you will be helping them out too.

Solution #2

Join a Support Group

Weight-loss support groups have been around for decades. You may have heard of one them.

It's called Weight Watchers.

Historically, people trying to lose weight have often been made to feel uncomfortable or embarrassed about sharing their goals or experiences with others. Being overweight or obese can be socially isolating, making it more difficult to connect. But Weight Watchers and other programs like Take Off Pounds Sensibly have embraced dieters and created a supportive forum for them to get educated, to be held accountable, and most of all to recognize that there are other people like them with similar concerns. It is not only empowering but also very effective.

Attending support groups is proven to result in weight loss, and more frequent attendance is directly correlated with more weight loss. The right support group will reinforce healthy practices, and self-weighing at meetings helps with accountability and also rewards persistence. In many ways, a support group can be many Solutions rolled into one. Find meetings in your local area at www.weightwatchers.com and www .tops.com, or ask about support groups offered at your hospital or primary care clinic.

But in-person support groups are not for everyone. They can involve travel and time out of your schedule, and there may be a weekly fee—and some people are not comfortable with public forums. Enter the Internet. It is relatively easy to find your own group online with people who know what you're going through. Websites like www.sparkpeople.com are a great place to start. Come and meet people who, like you, are trying to find their own solutions.

Solution #3

Use Automated Reminders

Using the evolving technology of social networking, millions of people are able to communicate information rapidly to a targeted audience with instant messages, status updates, and tweets. Friends use social networking to keep in touch, thought leaders use it to educate or influence people, and others use it to get information and updates about airline cancellations, sporting events, and breaking news.

One clever and effective use of instant messaging—text messaging in particular—is to help lose weight. This has been explored in multiple research studies. One study found that a weekly text about healthy eating, exercise, and beneficial lifestyle changes was associated with an *additional* weight loss of one pound per month. People who receive health texts are on average active for two hours more per week. And—to answer the obvious question—they don't find it annoying! Participants enjoy the reminders and consider them a helpful adjunct to their other weight-loss efforts.

Your first and most effective texting option is to text yourself. This way you choose the types of reminders you want to receive. You know what motivates you, and you also know where you might have some difficulties. Sending yourself an exercise reminder that coincides with your commute home or a "Get out of the candy dish!" reminder while you are at the office will make a real impact. Automated reminders can take lots of different shapes. Consider texting, tweeting, or e-mail. Services like www.ohdontforget.com provide free texts; www.tweetlater.com teaches you how to use Twitter to schedule reminder tweets; and Google Calendar provides possibly the best free and integrated system for sending yourself automated text messages and e-mail reminders up to one month in advance. Try any of these services and make mindfulness part of your every day.

Solution #4

Tatango!

Setting up your own text messaging system can take a small time investment right at the beginning. But what happens if you and a group of friends, teammates, or work colleagues want to do it together? I found a great service called Tatango that allows you to send group text messages as often as you like, for a small fee. It is incredibly easy to use, and gives you the flexibility to make your health journey a group effort. You can invite anyone to join your group, and if you no longer wish to send or receive messages, you can turn it off anytime. The cool thing about Tatango is that an unlimited number of people can join your group, so feel free to share this Solution with a friend. Check it out at www.tatango.com.

Solution #5

Get a Commitment from Your Significant Other

Unless you were lucky enough to have Richard Simmons as your justice of the peace, you may not have considered the role that a boyfriend, girlfriend, spouse, or significant other can play in helping you lose weight. When someone in your life takes an active interest in your diet or your health, it can make a huge difference in reaching your goals.

Get your significant other actively involved. That is what partners are supposed to do: support each other. There is nothing more frustrating than sitting down to a bowl of fruit while your significant other slathers butter on a slice of bacon and asks you to pass the half-and-half. Arguably, your weight loss benefits your partner, regardless of whether you are doing it to look better in your skivvies or to get off your blood pressure medication so that you can stick around for a few more decades. You both win if you get healthy—and he or she may actually get healthier too.

Research shows that spouses of dieters lose weight consistently even without meaning to. In fact, several studies show weight loss of *at least five pounds*. And the more frequently couples eat meals together, the more weight they lose as well.

So have a serious conversation with your significant other *today*. Frame the discussion around your goals and how you believe that you can reach them *together*. Share your Solutions and your plan, and get him or her on board. If you really want a commitment, get it on paper and sign a contract—it's time to renew those vows.

Solution #6

Find a Weight-Loss Buddy

Everyone needs a buddy. Because a buddy can be more than a friend or a setup for a bad movie about a cop and his dog. A buddy can be a Solution.

The purpose of a weight-loss buddy, diet buddy, or exercise buddy is to travel with you, literally or even just virtually, on this journey to a healthier life. But this is not a passive relationship. Your buddy can get you out of bed at five in the morning to go for a run, join you for lunch and keep you away from the deep-fried potato skins, or just be there for you online or on the telephone.

Remember, your buddy doesn't even need to be a friend or a spouse. You can meet a buddy on the Web or in a support group, or just by chance in a gym class or at a meeting. You know you have found a buddy once you recognize that you have similar goals and want to reach them together.

Buddies work because buddies make *you* work. And vice versa. You are more likely to have success with your weight-loss plan if you involve someone else and can help make him or her successful too. People with weight-loss buddies are proven to lose more weight than people who go it alone. For you to get the best benefit, your partner has to be right there in this with you. It turns out that it is a lot harder to be inspired by a normal-weight person than it is by an overweight person who *wants* to be normal weight.

Find a buddy in person or online. One-on-one or group buddies work with similar success. If you are looking for an Internet connection, some popular sites include www.webmd.com and www.medhelp.org (I admit it, I'm biased!). You can also check out www.weightlossbuddy .com, www.weightcircles.com, and www.diet.com for more ideas.

Solution #7

Follow People Who Inspire You on Twitter

Twitter is a strange beast—you either get it or you don't. But if you are willing to try something new, open a free account at www.twitter.com. The concept is simple. You post short messages or observations called tweets and have the ability to link to things online you find interesting and informative as well as add photos and videos that you take yourself. But the real value may be in how you can establish a connection with other people who interest you. You can do a quick search for "diet," "weight loss," "fitness," or any number of key words and easily find yourself on the other end of a surprisingly personal exchange in which you can become part of someone else's journey or learn facts or tricks to keep yours on the right track. You can follow doctors, exercise physiologists, and nutritionists, as well as people who are trying to make a difference in their own lives. And, yes, you can follow Ashton Kutcher too. It's free and worth a try. Check out my profile to get a sense of how it works at www.twitter.com/jamesbeckerman. I tweet about heart disease, diet, and healthy living, and I love following interesting people from all kinds of backgrounds. If you decide to follow me, send me a message and let me know you have read the book—I will be sure to follow you back!

Solution #8

Become Someone Else's Coach

Helping other people is not only the right thing to do, but it also helps you to view your own issues and challenges in proper context. Losing weight is hard enough, especially in a bubble. This is why I recommend that you involve other people in your journey, whether by blogging, following others on Twitter, joining a support group, or committing to a weight-loss buddy. But another option that many people do not think about is coaching.

Life coaching and diet coaching have grown in popularity over the past few years, especially with courses available online. Although training is a plus, less formal relationships can be just as helpful for you. Even though you may have had difficulty with your own weight in the past, this does not mean that you can't mentor someone else. It is not a case of "Those who can't do, teach" but rather of "Those who have been there can share their mistakes and their successes."

Case in point: One of my favorite diet bloggers is Shaun Chavis, who writes a blog at www.health.com. My favorite post of hers is called "I'm a 225-Pound Weight-Loss Editor. Get Over It." Shaun makes a great point that people with diabetes or cancer are often sought for their expertise and perspectives on their condition, but people with weight struggles are not usually considered authorities on the subject. Who is the better mentor? Someone who has always been thin and doesn't actively think about weight loss, or someone who is battling the bulge every day, who follows the latest research and insights, and who is just as frustrated as you are? It is easier to listen to a coach or mentor when you believe the person has empathy for what you are experiencing.

There are multiple avenues to becoming a coach. If you are interested in doing it professionally, you can find coursework online and in person—check out Coach U at www.coachinc.com. Making a business out of taking care of people is incredibly satisfying—trust me on that. But if you are interested in a less formal relationship, consider advertising your services on message boards or even Craigslist. Talk to the friends with whom you commiserate, and mention the idea of one coaching the other to turn your frustrations into something positive. You can still keep it personal but provide honesty and constructive advice. After all, you've been there, or you *are* there right now. Coaching someone else will force you to look inward as well and think more carefully about the decisions *you* make. If someone else is counting on you, you can't help but try to be more accountable to yourself too.

Solution #9

Blog

Blogs have been around for the past decade, but have skyrocketed in popularity over the last couple of years. People blog about everything. Blogging is informative, opinionated, and occasionally annoying, but all blogs share a common thread: catharsis. Blogging is the epitome of the open playing field, and it allows you to express yourself in a way that was not previously available. And while people sometimes equate blogging with writing in a diary, the blogging platform implies that you are willing to put yourself out there and make your dirty laundry public. But anonymously, if you like.

The first blog about weight loss probably appeared on the second day of blogging history. Given the challenges of dieting and the inevitable frustrations, blogging provides a great outlet for your angst, and it actually encourages you to explore your greatest difficulties while at the same time allowing you to highlight your successes. And because blogs invite commentary, you get feedback (whether positive or negative) and are somehow accountable to your readers—even if that means only your mother.

You can start a blog for free; popular platforms include www.blogger.com and www.wordpress.com. They are surprisingly easy to use—you can be on your way in just a couple of minutes. Write about anything you like, from recipes that have worked out well for you to tricks that you find helpful to annoyances that you know other people will relate to.

Another great feature of blogs is that you can subscribe to them, so even if you are not interested in chronicling your own experiences, you can subscribe to other people's blogs and be notified by e-mail when they update them. Here are some interesting weight-loss blogs to get you started.

www.amerrylife.com
www.bodyforwife.com
www.dietgirl.org
www.fertilehealthy.com/blog
www.fitbottomedgirls.blogspot.com
www.fitbymy50th.blogspot.com
www.marksdailyapple.com
www.mizfitonline.com
www.priorfatgirl.com
www.ronisweigh.com
www.whoatemyblog.com

And don't forget www.jamesbeckerman.com! If you start your own blog, please leave me a comment and let me know so that I can follow your progress.

Solution #10

Call Your Doctor

Before you start any serious weight-loss plan, you really should speak with your doctor. Even though I am a cardiologist and this book makes every attempt to offer sound, healthful ideas, it is very important to let your doctor know what you are up to. It is easy to forget that medications can impact what type of diet you should be following, and your doctor may also have concerns about your level of activity if you have heart or lung disease.

Medical conditions like hypothyroidism, Cushing's syndrome, and polycystic ovarian syndrome may cause weight gain, so make sure that you have been checked for possible health problems and are receiving any treatment that may be indicated. It is also true that some of the medicines that doctors prescribe are associated with weight gain. If you are on multiple medications, it is a good idea to begin a dialogue with your health care provider about potential side effects that could be hindering your weight-loss efforts. There are often alternative medicines that can be prescribed. Common offenders may include corticosteroids, some antidepressants and antipsychotics, and migraine and seizure medicines, as well as some medicines for treating high blood pressure and diabetes. If you are on any of these, do not stop them without discussing this first with your doctor and identifying possible substitutions.

There is another discussion that some people should have with their physician, especially when embarking on a diet. It's about depression. Depression impacts one in eight individuals, making it one of the most common medical conditions in the world. When diagnosed and treated appropriately, most people experience a substantial benefit. But like many medical conditions, depression can be uncomfortably silent, and is often underdiagnosed. Whereas almost anyone can recognize when someone is overweight, physicians and nonphysicians alike often fail to recognize depression. Nonpsychiatrist physicians miss the diagnosis over half the time—which means that over half of people with depression who seek medical care may not be getting the care that they need.

This is very humbling from a physician's perspective. Part of the challenge of diagnosing depression is interpreting symptoms in the context of other complex medical problems. For example, many people with heart disease experience either fatigue or a lack of motivation to do certain things because of concerns about exacerbating their symptoms. But in some individuals this can also be a manifestation of depression.

We know that heart disease can be associated with depression, and some studies suggest that treatment of depression may result in better clinical outcomes. The same can be said for the effect on weight. Treating depression in overweight individuals can certainly result in improvement in their quality of life. But you may also be wondering whether it might help them lose weight as well. If this is a concern of yours, it might be just one more reason to call your doctor, set up an appointment, and get the treatment you may need.

We already know that weight gain can be a marker for depression, particularly in people who are already overweight. There is a link between depression and unhealthy lifestyle habits. The relationship has been examined in research studies that have used antidepressant medication to treat depression, with an eye toward its impact on weight loss. And overall the data are encouraging. The drug buproprion has been found to be associated with a weight loss of about six pounds in six months. Sertraline was associated with a more modest weight loss of one to two pounds in two to four months. Fluoxetine was associated with a five-pound weight loss in about six months. It is important to stress, however, that these antidepressant drugs are appropriate for individuals with depression, not just for use in weight-loss. In some studies higher doses have been used than are typically used for depression alone, and there are concerns about long-term safety.

Medications are not necessarily for everybody. There are other options, including therapy. An exciting current clinical trial is examining the impact of therapy on weight loss as compared to standard weight-loss treatment alone. It will be a two-year study, and I hope that it will provide some additional possibilities. Results from prior studies are encouraging; one study of cognitive therapy found a significant weight-loss result, and people felt better about themselves too.

Bottom line, taking care of yourself means looking after everything, from above your collar to what's hanging over your belt. And there may be some connections there that even your doctor does not completely understand. Treatment of one may actually help in treating the other.

Solution #11

Weigh Yourself Daily

Many of the most effective weight-loss Solutions are not directives to do exercise or eat less. Things like wearing a pedometer, keeping a food diary, and giving yourself financial incentives (just you wait . . .) do not actually burn calories. But they do motivate you and keep you thinking about what you are trying to accomplish. You then change behavior, and eventually you no longer need them.

Some people debate about whether dieters should weigh themselves. This is because dieters often fear the scale. While it can be a measure of success, it is also a reminder that this is not easy. Some feel that unless they are making huge progress between weigh-ins, frequent weighing will only demotivate them. But the scientific data suggest that this behavior greatly improves one's chances of losing weight.

One study actually found that weighing yourself more frequently is associated with greater weight loss than weighing yourself only periodically. Daily weigh-ins were associated with double the weight loss of weekly ones, whereas people who did not weigh themselves at all *gained* weight during the period of time covered by the study. In fact, people who changed their weighing behavior during the study actually gained or lost weight depending on whether they decreased or increased their frequency of weighing themselves.

Weighing yourself daily lets you know when things may be going off track so that you can make small changes, even day to day, rather than realizing after a month that you have gained seven pounds and feel that you need to make drastic changes to get back to where you want to be. And we know that drastic changes often backfire.

The benefits of daily weigh-ins have also been highlighted in studies of two particularly sensitive times for gaining weight quickly—the holidays and starting college. One study found that people gained five times more weight during the holidays than in a typical week, but those who weighed themselves daily actually lost weight during the same period of time. Similarly, several studies have found that college freshmen who weighed themselves daily avoided the "freshman fifteen" as compared to students who did not weigh themselves at all.

Some opponents of this strategy argue that such frequent weighing can be stressful and lead people to focus too much on their weight. This is an interesting point that cannot be ignored, and it is especially applicable to individuals with eating disorders or an unhealthy and unrealistic self-image. But for those individuals who are overweight or obese and who are actively trying to lose weight in a healthy, safe manner, research supports daily weighing. And it is encouraging to know that large-scale studies have found that frequent self-weighing has no association with becoming depressed, but is instead associated with more willpower and restraint.

Solution #12

Warm Up

Calisthenics are possibly the easiest form of exercise to undertake anytime or anywhere—all you need is you. No weights. No equipment. A carpet is helpful, as are some forgiving downstairs neighbors, but neither is essential. And the best part is that you can start *today*.

You might associate calisthenics with the stretching exercises that high school students perform prior to engaging in more competitive sports. But calisthenics have a long history; they were originally developed in the 1800s to increase muscle strength by using the body's own weight for resistance. And they still work.

Calisthenics include a variety of exercises that you can do in your own home. Remember that exercises that develop lean muscle mass increase your metabolism and help you burn calories even when you are not exercising. And calisthenics can burn 300 to 600 calories per hour, depending on your body weight and how vigorously you do them. Start with a reasonable goal, such as twenty minutes a day. Do twenty repetitions of each of the following exercises twice a day. You can divide them into morning and evening rituals, or you can do one after another to get yourself started in the morning. You can do them while you watch television. You can also incorporate them into other forms of aerobic exercise, like running or walking, for an even greater burn. Be flexible.

Warm-up Solution	What You Do
Sit-ups	Lie with your back on the floor, with knees bent and feet planted on the floor. Bring your chest to your knees without using your arms or hands for support.
Crunches	Similar to sit-ups, but done without bringing your chest all the way to your knees. Concentrate on using your abdominal muscles to bring your shoulder blades off the floor.
Push-ups	Lie facedown on the floor, with the palms of your hands and your toes touching the floor. Push with your hands and extend your arms so that you bring yourself up off the floor. You can allow your knees to touch the floor if you need to.
Squats	Stand with your back straight and your feet about shoulder width apart. Keeping your back straight and facing forward, bend your knees all the way. Then return to a standing position without bending forward.
Calf raises	Stand on your toes, and then slowly return your heels to the floor.
Jumping jacks	Stand with your arms at your sides and your feet together. Jump and land with your legs spread wide as you clap your hands over your head. Then return to your original position.

Solution #13

Keep a Food Diary

You are what you eat. But do you *remember* what you eat? Whenever I sit down with a patient and begin a conversation about weight loss, I always start things off by asking, "Can you tell me what you ate yesterday?" Men will look at their wives for direction, and women look at the floor or out the window for clarification.

Socrates famously said, "The unexamined life is not worth living." In the present context we might say, "The unexamined diet is not working." While food diaries probably have not been around for as long as the words of Socrates, they can be traced at least as far back as the Victorian era, when London actor John Pritt Harley was gracing the stage of the Princess's Theatre on Oxford Street. His January 4, 1858, entry details a day in his life.

> Rehearsal at two, home to dinner at four. Roast beef, potato, biscuit, cheese, ale, port, and sherry. Tea at seven. Left letter of excuse and card at J. Cooke's on having to decline dining with him tomorrow. Home at ten, supped at eleven, cold roast beef, biscuit, cheese, ale, gin and water. Read Spectator to Betsy. Bed at one.

Not many vegetables in those days. But one thing we do know about John Pritt Harley is that his nickname, "Fat Jack," was something of a misnomer—he was a tall and skinny guy. Did his food diary have something to do with that?

Research studies have demonstrated that a food diary is the *single most effective strategy* for losing weight in the long term. People who keep a food diary can experience double the weight loss of people who go it alone. It may be that paying attention to those late-night snacks, extra fries, and second helpings may result in eating fewer of them. A sample food diary is presented on the following page. Make some copies to get yourself started.

THE FLEX DIET FOOD DIARY

BREAKFAST time _____
Food _____
_____
_____
_____

Beverage _____

LUNCH time _____
Food _____
_____
_____
_____
_____

Beverage _____

DINNER time _____
Food _____
_____
_____
_____

Beverage _____

SNACKS (with times)
_____
_____
_____
_____

Solution #14

Drink Six Glasses of Water a Day

Water is essential for your good health. It keeps your blood flowing, provides cushioning for your joints, and transports nutrients into and waste out of cells. But I want to dispel the myth that you need to drink eight large glasses of water each day. This recommendation is widely shared in health newsletters, on blogs, and by physicians, but without much evidence to support it. Kidney specialists would argue that you need only about a liter of water per day to make up for losses—that's about four eight-ounce glasses. We consume just about that in food alone, suggesting that many people could get by safely without drinking any additional fluids. Of course, fluid losses will vary, depending on climate, your level of activity, and even—if you are a man—your prostate. The straight dope on water is that you should drink it when you are thirsty.

Except if you want to lose weight. Simply put, water takes up space. And if you are not drinking it, you might be drinking or eating something else with a lot of calories. Water can make you feel full and can function as an appetite suppressant. Researchers have found that drinking four to six glasses a day is associated with weight loss. Interestingly, drinking even two glasses of water a day will speed up your metabolism and help you burn calories faster. Thirsty? Keeping a bottle of water at your desk or drinking a glass before each meal is a great way to easily incorporate it into your day.

Solution #15

Take a Multivitamin

About half of all Americans take a multivitamin on a regular basis. But if you look at the numbers, you will find that overweight and obese individuals are less likely to take vitamins than normal-weight individuals. This correlation deserves further attention.

Taking a daily multivitamin is a cheap and safe intervention. But

Supplements

Supplements are playing an increasing role in the diet world, but it is important to consider carefully what you are taking, and why. One of the challenges of choosing supplements is that a lack of regulation makes it easy for manufacturers and marketers to make completely false and unsubstantiated claims about useless or even dangerous products. Add a celebrity endorsement or a full-page ad in a magazine, and even the most discriminating consumer can be duped. With the promise of easy weight loss, supplements make dieters an easy target for exploitation. It is important to review which supplements are safe and which are to be avoided. Also keep in mind that no supplement is a substitute for a healthy diet and exercise. A multivitamin is just one of many Solutions. And before you start taking anything, let your doctor know.

does it have much benefit? Some would argue that as long as you are getting adequate nourishment, supplements are not necessary. But research shows that overweight and obese people are at risk for deficiencies in a number of nutrients, including vitamin C, vitamin D, vitamin E, folate, alpha-carotene, beta-carotene, beta-cryptoxanthin, lutein, lycopene, zeaxanthin, total carotenoids, and selenium. One assumption is that overweight people eat too much junk food that is low in nutrients, but it seems more likely that excess weight alters the absorption and metabolism of vitamins. Overweight people can become vitamin deficient even if they are consuming a diet similar to that of people of normal weight. It is even possible that the brain detects this relative deficiency and guides overweight people to eat more in order to make up for it.

So the next question is whether supplementing with a multivitamin can not only help with deficiencies, but can also help with weight loss. Preliminary studies suggest that taking a multivitamin is associated with a decrease in appetite as well as an increased sensation of being full after eating—and both are moves in the right direction. Other studies suggest that a multivitamin may also be associated with modest weight loss. For example, a long-term study found that taking a multivitamin high in chromium was associated with a three-pound weight loss over time, whereas those people not taking any vitamins gained ten pounds in the same time frame.

You do not need to look far to find an inexpensive general multivitamin. Brands like Centrum and One A Day have a good reputation for accurate labeling and freedom from impurities. A supplement should be taken in addition to a healthy diet, not instead of one. But remember that just because a supplement can be beneficial does not mean that you should take ten of the tablets daily. There is a risk of oversupplementing, especially with vitamin A. One A day means just once a day.

Solution #16

Get Your Calcium

Few people get the recommended daily amount of calcium. Concerns about bone loss and fractures lead many older women to take a supplement, especially after menopause. And as with most things, prevention is a more effective tactic than addressing the problem once it has occurred.

Scientists have been looking at calcium for many years and have uncovered some interesting information about calcium deficiency and body weight. It turns out that people low in calcium tend to be more overweight. This has led researchers to examine the impact of supplementing calcium in overweight people to see what happens.

One study gave obese women who were getting less than 600 milligrams of calcium a day a 1,200-milligram supplement or a placebo. Over the course of fifteen weeks, those in the calcium-supplement group lost an average of ten pounds more than those in the placebo group. The participants taking calcium had less belly fat, more lean muscle mass, and better cholesterol levels after just a few weeks.

Scientists hypothesize that when you are low in calcium, your brain tells you to consume more calcium-containing items, many of which are high in calories and fat. Others believe that calcium supplementation helps the body break down fat more effectively. Studies suggest that dairy sources may also be effective; this may be because dairy calories are being substituted for other foods that may not be as beneficial, like soda.

Most Americans do not get the amount of calcium they need every day. It is recommended that both men and premenopausal women get at least 1,000 milligrams. If you are pregnant or postmenopausal, talk to your doctor about specific recommendations, which are higher. And while you're at it, ask your doctor to check your vitamin D levels too—vitamin D deficiency has been shown to be associated with many chronic health problems. You can get your daily 1,000 milligrams of calcium by taking one tablet of Tums Ultra 1000 Maximum Strength twice a day with food—calcium is absorbed better in divided doses. If you experience constipation or are taking medication for acid reflux, consider taking calcium citrate—as in Citracal—instead. Avoid "natural" calcium supplements such as oyster-shell calcium or bone meal that are less regulated and may contain lead.

Solution #17

Consider Taking Fish Oil

Whereas there is a wealth of data supporting the use of fish oil to improve cardiovascular health, using fish oil to maintain a healthy weight is an exciting new area of exploration. One theory holds that fish oil improves blood vessel function and therefore blood *flow* to exercising muscles, resulting in more efficient metabolism of fat during exercise. This means weight-loss. And fish oil supplements may provide even additional weight loss benefits as compared to actually eating fish. Findings also suggest that combining a fish oil supplement with regular exercise can be more effective for weight loss than either of these interventions attempted alone. Pharmaceutical companies and supplement manufacturers are now offering purified fish oil in capsules that are well tolerated and have very limited interactions with medication.

The beneficial components of fish oil are the omega-3 fatty acids, and there are three types. EPA (eicosapentaenoic acid) and DHA (docosahexaenoic acid) are the "long-chain" forms found in fish and fish oil. ALA (alpha-linolenic acid) is a "short-chain" form found in plant

sources like walnuts, flaxseed, and canola and soybean oils, and is probably less effective because relatively little is converted to the more active
EPA and DHA forms. Consuming up to two grams daily of EPA and
DHA should be safe for most people, but more than this may increase
bleeding risks, and should be done only under a doctor's supervision.

Older adults remember being given a tablespoon of cod liver oil for
medicinal purposes, but this is not currently recommended because of
potential risks related to contaminants as well as the cumulative effects
of too much vitamin A. Similarly, you should look for fish oil supplement brands that have a good track record for purifying the oil to meet
safety standards. Nature's Bounty, GNC, and CVS Pharmacy are some
good examples. Check out the Environmental Defense Fund's website
(www.edf.org) for safe possibilities in your area.

The most commonly cited side effects include burping or a fishy af-
tertaste. Taking the capsules with meals and keeping them in the refrigerator have been shown to reduce side effects significantly. Fish oil may
increase the risk of bleeding, particularly in people on blood thinners,
so it's important to discuss it with your own doctor. And remember, the
idea is not to enjoy a fish oil supplement with a bag of chips, but to incorporate it into a healthier diet. Take two grams a day.

Solution #18

Look into Probiotics

Between H1N1 epidemics and just good manners, we are so condi-
tioned to cover our mouths and wash our hands when we sneeze that
it is easy to think that all microorganisms, including bacteria, are to be
avoided. But probiotics are friendly bacteria that you should actually get
to know a little bit better.

We already know that bacteria and other microorganisms are everywhere, from the surface of our skin to the inside of our intestines. But
some are healthier for us than others. Whereas antibiotics are medications we use to kill germs, probiotics are carefully isolated bacteria and
yeasts that help to restore the normal balance of microorganisms in the

intestinal tract. Probiotics crowd out germs that are not good for us and also may foster an environment in which the bad guys cannot thrive.

Probiotics have been used for years, primarily for relieving gastrointestinal problems. New data suggest that they may also be helpful for weight loss. Two very different populations have recently been studied: mothers who had just given birth, and obese individuals who had undergone gastric bypass surgery. In both groups, subjects given probiotics experienced significant weight loss as compared to the people who just got placebos.

Most probiotics used in supplements or in food are bacteria from the *Lactobacillus* and *Bifidobacterium lactis* species. They can be found in yogurt (like Dannon's Activia), cheese (like Kraft's Knudsen LiveActive), fermented or unfermented milk (like Bio-K+ CL1285 fermented milk), miso, and some soy beverages. But they are also sold in capsules and powders (like those from Culturelle) that you can find at your local pharmacy. They are not medicines and are not supervised by the Food and Drug Administration. There are multiple brands and types available. Probiotics may contain many types of bacteria, so there are no set dosages. Taking at least two billion live cells daily is typically recommended. Most scientists and health care providers believe that probiotics are safe, but make sure you discuss them with your own doctor.

Solution #19

Try Taking Whey Protein After Exercise

Whey protein is a natural part of dairy foods like milk, cottage cheese, and yogurt. It is also widely available as a powdered supplement that can be made into a shake. Whey protein can play an interesting role in a weight-loss program, particularly when incorporated into a weight-lifting routine.

Whey protein is digested very quickly by the body, which means that it can be used more quickly than other forms of nutrition—even other types of protein. The supplemental form is also very low in other types of calories, like those from carbohydrates or fat, which means that if you consume it after weight-bearing exercise, it will go straight to your muscles.

While it is true that whey protein alone will not make you lose weight, it can help change your body composition when combined with lifting weights. The protein helps to repair and build muscle while you burn calories to reduce fat. One study found that people taking a whey protein supplement lost three pounds more body fat than those in the control group. While it may be best to use whey protein supplement as an exercise-recovery drink within thirty minutes of exercise, you can also have a shake as an occasional meal replacement or substitute one for your regular afternoon snack. Look for whey protein supplements without any additional ingredients, and avoid them if you are allergic to milk or are taking antibiotics. Consider brands like 100% Whey Protein, Elite Whey Protein Isolate, Pure Whey Protein Stack, and Complete Whey. Information for proper dosing is not readily available, but some studies recommend one gram per kilogram of body weight for each serving. If you experience headaches or bloating, you are taking too much.

No-lutions

The most commonly advertised supplements are unfortunately the ones that are to be avoided. They are not well supported by scientific evidence, and in some cases they can be dangerous. They are not Solutions—they're *No*-lutions and should not be a part of the Flex Diet.

Bitter Orange

When ephedra was banned because of increased risk of heart attacks and strokes, some supplement manufacturers turned to other stimulants with similar profiles as "natural" supplement alternatives. Bitter orange is one of those stimulants. Derived from the fruit of the tree *Citrus aurantium*, bitter orange has gained popularity because of its similarities to ephedra without the legal entanglements. Unfortunately, its similarities likely extend into its risk profile. Bitter orange contains synephrine, a compound very similar to ephedrine that constricts blood vessels and consequently increases heart rate and blood pressure. It is suspected to be as dangerous as ephedra, and case reports have linked it to strokes and angina. And if that doesn't convince you not to use it, you should note that there is not any evidence to suggest that it is an effective weight-loss supplement. Bitter indeed.

Apple Cider Vinegar

Apple cider vinegar has been touted as a next-generation weight-loss supplement that is natural and safe. Unfortunately, there is little evidence to support its use. While you would like to think that fifty years of users could not be wrong, data have not shown that apple cider vinegar will help you lose weight. Much of the excitement around it is based upon a single study of twelve individuals who felt more full after eating small amounts of vinegar on bread. Delicious. But one study of twelve people who felt full does not substantiate claims about significant weight loss.

There are other potential benefits, however, that should not be ignored. Some small, preliminary studies have suggested that apple cider vinegar may play a role in lowering blood sugar in diabetics, lowering cholesterol, and potentially lowering blood pressure. These studies have involved rats or just a handful of people and thus are far from conclusive.

Before you start dousing yourself in the stuff, please keep in mind that vinegar is very acidic and can wreak havoc on your digestive system and bones if not taken under proper medical supervision. It can also interact with medication that you might be taking for high blood pressure or diabetes. And if you take it in its supplement form, you don't really know what you are getting. One chemical analysis of apple cider vinegar supplements even raised the question of whether the supplements contained any vinegar at all. Eat it on a salad if you enjoy it, but avoid it as a supplement until more research is available.

Acai Berry

The last time a small piece of fruit got so many people in trouble, palm fronds were in style and snake oil salesmen were actually serpents. Times have changed, but unsubstantiated claims and false advertising have not. Enter the acai berry, diet fruit to the stars and ubiquitous Internet pop-up ad. It is hard to get anything done online these days without coming upon a testimonial about how pills, smoothies, and juices derived from this innocuous little berry have changed someone's life for the better. And it can be yours for just one low price. . . .

The acai berry is a grape-sized dark-colored fruit eaten commonly in Brazil as well as other countries in the Amazon region. While research would support claims that it has antioxidant properties, it is not as potent as grapes, strawberries, or even red wine. Most important, no published study has ever demonstrated that it has any significant effect on weight loss, let alone health benefits of any kind that would not be expected from eating other fruits. Although it is touted as a "superfood," its supporters are hard pressed to provide convincing scientific data that there is anything super about it. Sorry to disappoint.

Guar Gum

Whereas dietary fiber has been demonstrated to contribute to healthy weight loss as well as protect against heart disease and some cancers, fiber in pill or powder form tends to be less effective. Guar gum is derived from the Indian cluster bean. Like beans, guar gum does absorb water, and this can result in a feeling of fullness. And also like beans, guar gum can lead to abdominal distress. Perhaps this is because it can absorb enough water to grow in size by ten or twenty times, leading to obstruction of the esophagus as well as the intestines. An extensive review of guar gum found no significant impact on weight loss as compared to placebo. It seems as though the only weight you could lose is what you lose while you are recovering from surgery after having a watermelon-sized ball of guar gum removed from your colon. Enjoy!

~~Hoodia~~

Well known to readers of magazine advertisements, hoodia is a weight-loss supplement with an interesting history. Hoodia is derived from a plant traditionally consumed by African Bushmen to ward off hunger, but it has gained celebrity *because of* celebrities throughout the rest of the world. Very small nonrandomized studies have suggested that it may live up to some of its claims as an appetite suppressant, but thorough research has not been performed to date. Pharmaceutical giant Pfizer purchased the rights to study hoodia's active ingredient, but returned those rights to a smaller laboratory a few years later. Not a good sign. In addition to concerns that hoodia supplements often do not actually contain hoodia (you can never know because the substance is not regulated), some studies suggest that hoodia can cause adverse effects on the liver and make life difficult for diabetics, pregnant women, the elderly, and children.

~~hCG~~

Human chorionic gonadotropin, or hCG, is a hormone found in the urine of pregnant women. Not my idea of a good starting point for a diet, but hCG injections are recommended in some diet programs. hCG stimulates ovulation and testosterone production. Its use is not scientifically supported for weight loss, and side effects include but are not limited to breast enlargement in men, fatigue, mood changes, swelling, and hair loss, not to mention the risks related to self-injection.

Solution #20

Wear a Pedometer

Walking is something that you do to get from point A to point B. But if you wear a pedometer while you are doing it, it becomes exercise. Multiple research studies have demonstrated that an informal walking exercise program guided by a pedometer results in weight loss, even without dietary interventions. It seems that the pedometer encourages you to walk with a daily goal in mind, and the presence of the pedometer on your belt serves as a reminder to keep moving.

Conceived by the Romans, imagined by Leonardo da Vinci, and invented by Thomas Jefferson, the pedometer counts the number of steps a person takes by detecting hip motion. Originally recognized for their potential military applications, pedometers are used today primarily for fitness purposes. Walking two thousand steps typically corresponds to about a mile. Experts generally recommend trying to reach a daily goal of ten thousand steps for optimal results.

Research indicates that wearing a pedometer is associated with losing weight. Having a daily goal, and keeping a step diary to record it, is associated with even more success. (It will take only a few seconds to add this information to the food diary you are already maintaining.) And longer-duration pedometer-based walking programs are associated with continued weight loss; participants in one study who wore a pedometer for one year lost over eight pounds.

Wearing a pedometer does not cramp your lifestyle or wardrobe significantly; pedometers are about the size of a pager and are simple to use. Wearing one can quickly be incorporated into your life *today*. Simple pedometers can be found in any sporting goods store. There are also pedometer applications available for the iPhone, as well as digital pedometers like the Fitbit Tracker and the Philips DirectLife Activity Monitor for the more technologically savvy. These may be more expensive, but they have fun features that may be worth the money.

Solution #21
Don't Use Exercise as a Punishment

This Solution is not about a particular way to take in healthy calories or burn them, and it's also not really about mindfulness. But it speaks to your philosophy about losing weight or just being healthy. Many of us think about weight loss and weight gain in terms of calories. It is a simple metric: 3,500 calories taken in equals a pound, and 3,500 calories out equals a pound. This straightforward math gets us thinking about calories almost like a currency that can be saved, spent, and bartered. But beware of calorie extortion.

We have all been there before. You have eaten a healthy meal, and then comes the question of dessert. As you look through the options, you are already starting to negotiate with yourself. What is that sundae worth? How many minutes on the treadmill if I eat the cheesecake? Sure, if there was a guarantee that you would be exercising forty-five minutes *extra* every time you drank a milkshake, then there would not be an issue. But the problem is that we are just not that trustworthy. The evening comes and goes, and there you are, frustrated as you lie in bed, knowing that you did not hold up your end of the bargain. And the dessert unfortunately *always* does.

This kind of pattern can lead to an unhealthy relationship with exercise in which it becomes a punishment for the foods we enjoy. This puts exercise in a negative light—and the last thing we need is another reason not to do it. Try not to deal with calories as currency on a day-to-day basis—remember that your goal is an overall healthy economy. Food and exercise can work together, but it is easier to think of them separately.

Snacks

Snacking is a Solution. But the difference between a snack in a weight-loss program and snacking on your own is that a planned snack can actually help you lose weight. The key is control. When you have set aside a little time in the midafternoon to get some needed energy, you satisfy your hunger and prevent spontaneous snacking later on. The choice of snack is key. Pick one of the seven snacks listed below to enjoy every day. You might find it easier to stick with the same one—a routine leaves less opportunity for rogue snacking later on. Research also suggests that minimizing variety may lead to more significant weight loss.

Solution #22

Almonds

Nuts like almonds are recommended for two nutritional qualities. First, they are an excellent source of monounsaturated fats. Not all fats are created equal. *Saturated fats* are bad for your cholesterol levels and they may increase your risk of developing heart disease; they are found in foods like red meat, butter, and coconut oil. *Trans fats* are even more dangerous—and unfortunately are often present in doughnuts, French fries, and baked goods. The healthier fats are *unsaturated;* they include monounsaturated fat, polyunsaturated fat, and omega-3 fatty acids (as in fish oil). Almonds are high in monounsaturated fats (only macadamia nuts and pecans have more). They may reduce your risk of developing coronary artery disease by significantly bringing down your LDL (low-density lipoprotein) cholesterol.

Nuts are also beneficial because of their low-glycemic-index rating. The glycemic index, or GI, is a ranking of carbohydrate foods according to their impact on your blood sugar levels. High levels are worse, and low levels better. Health risks related to high-glycemic foods include diabetes, heart disease, and obesity.

Researchers have linked the low GI of almonds to their potential for promoting healthy weight. Adding extra daily calories in the form of almonds does not change weight significantly, and when you enjoy an almond snack instead of a high-carbohydrate snack like crackers or popcorn, you will tend to lose weight.

Compared to other nuts, almonds are highest in protein and vitamins, and they are the best researched in terms of a beneficial effect on weight loss. Stick to the unsalted ones to avoid bumping up your blood pressure in the process. Eat about twenty (an ounce) for a substantial snack. Maisie Jane's and Blue Diamond are two brands that package almonds in individual-serving sizes to make things even easier for you.

Almond butter is another great way to enjoy almonds, and it can be used as a substitute for peanut butter. Whereas peanut butter may have salt, sugar, and other additives, almond butter is essentially just crushed almonds. Two ounces of almond butter should provide a benefit similar to that of about twenty whole almonds. While unsweetened almond "milk" is a great lower-calorie alternative to cow's milk, you would have to drink at least four glasses a day to get the same benefit as you would from a handful of almonds.

Solution? Go nuts.

Solution #23

Apples

Although we all know that an apple a day can keep the doctor away, many of us do not eat fruit at all, unless it accompanies ice cream and hot fudge. Some dieters perceive fruit as too high in sugar to be a healthy weight-loss snack. While fruit does have higher sugar levels than some other snack foods, it has some significant advantages—as listed below—that should also be considered.

1. **High in nutrients.** Fruit is a great source of Vitamin A and Vitamin C.

2. **High in fiber.** Fruit helps keep you fuller for longer.

3. **Low in sodium.** You might not care, but your cardiologist will be happy.

4. **Low on the glycemic index.** The sugars in fruit are broken down slowly as compared to those in fruit juice, which generally has a higher GI and raises blood sugar more quickly.

5. **Low in calories.** Compared to other snacks, fruit provides lower calorie content in a pretty substantial serving size. *Energy density* is the concept that in a given volume of a food there is a specific number of calories, as determined by the food's water, fiber, and fat content. Larger-portion foods with

fewer calories are low in energy density, and make great weight-loss snacks because they fill you up, whereas smaller-portion foods with lots of calories—like chocolate—are not the best choices.

Not only is fruit good for you, but it is proven to help you lose weight. When people eat fruit like apples or pears instead of eating the same number of calories in cookies or other snacks, they lose weight. Despite having similar amounts of fiber and calories, fruit and cookies differ in energy density, which impacts fullness and ultimately influences what else you choose to eat over the course of the day. The weight reduction is often accompanied by improvements in cholesterol and blood sugar levels as well.

Eat a piece of fruit as an afternoon snack. Apples and pears have the best evidence as weight-loss foods, but substituting a banana or an orange is acceptable. Try eating at least two pieces of fruit a day, whether for your lunchtime dessert, as a snack, or during the evening commute home. Having a bowl of fruit in your kitchen or at your desk is a great way to remind yourself to grab some even when you are busy. Another great trick is to grab an apple on your way out to meet people for dinner—it keeps you away from the breadbasket and freshens your breath too.

Solution #24

Grapes

Grapes are a great snack at any time of day. They satisfy your sweet tooth, and because of their high water content they make you feel full. And one grape has only about 2 calories—you can enjoy your snack with relative abandon and not feel guilty about it. Most weight-loss plans, including the Flex Diet, recommend against snacking at night, but if you just have to have a snack while watching Letterman, try some grapes instead of ice cream or chips. You can put them in the freezer for an hour before you eat them to make them seem more like candy, or even drizzle a tiny bit of honey over them to bring out the flavor. And keep them on the stalk instead of placing them individually in a bowl—it will take just a little bit longer to finish them and you will feel you've had a more substantial snack.

Solution #25

Greek Yogurt

You may already be taking a calcium supplement. But consuming more dairy calcium is also associated with doubling weight loss in some studies, even when people are not actively reducing their calorie intake. Skim or nonfat dairy foods are often recommended, but many people complain that nonfat dairy products just don't taste as good as their full-fat counterparts. Greek yogurt to the rescue.

Greek yogurt is basically regular yogurt that has gone through a strainer. It has a much creamier texture and a delicious taste without the runny consistency that sends people straight to the ice cream counter instead. Nonfat and low-fat options are widely available. Here is a comparison between Greek yogurt (Fage Total 0%) and regular yogurt (Dannon All Natural Nonfat Plain), with nutritional information given per ounce. The Greek yogurt has almost double the protein content, which helps satisfy your hunger. Individual serving sizes make figuring out portions easy—or just spoon yourself a cupful.

YOGURT (1 ounce)	CALORIES	FAT (g)	SUGAR (g)	PROTEIN (g)
Fage Total 100%	15	0	1	2.5
Dannon Nonfat Plain	13	0	2	1.5

Another advantage of Greek yogurt is its versatility. It works well in both sweet and savory dishes, and it can easily be incorporated into snacks, smoothies, desserts, and regular meals, especially breakfast. Add lemon juice, garlic, and a bit of thyme to make tzatziki, or just a touch of sugar-free syrup and a few almonds for a snack or dessert. Use it as a substitute for sour cream, or to thicken smoothies, and even get more mileage out of peanut butter by mixing the two together.

Solution #26
Flaxseeds

A relatively new diet concept is the "superfood." Guests on daytime talk shows extol the virtues of a particular berry or spice, and then the supplement manufacturers hawk "extracts" and "concentrates" on the Internet a few hours later. The truth is that there is no single food that does it all. But flaxseed comes pretty close.

These tiny seeds have been eaten for thousands of years, and now are incorporated into foods like crackers, oatmeal, and waffles. Flaxseed is rich in omega-3 fatty acids, antioxidants, and fiber, which make it a great food to incorporate into a weight-loss program. It has also been suggested that flaxseed can reduce your risk of heart disease, cancer, and diabetes, not to mention hot flashes. Sounds pretty super, doesn't it?

Flaxseed is recommended for dieters because it decreases the digestibility (and absorption) of fat. This means that like other high-fiber foods, flaxseed may help you actually take in less fat from the other foods you normally eat. Ground flaxseed appears to be more beneficial than flaxseed oil alone. The optimal "dose" is still uncertain, but many experts agree that one to two tablespoons of ground flaxseed a day is sufficient to yield benefits. You can spoon it up and wash it down with some water, or add it to yogurt for an afternoon snack.

When you buy flaxseed at the supermarket, it is best to buy whole seeds because they last longer. If you buy ground seeds or grind the seeds yourself (a coffee bean grinder works well), you can store the flaxseed in the freezer for up to a year. You can then add it to foods you normally eat, like oatmeal or soups, and you can also add it to casseroles and stews without significantly changing the taste. Another trick is to use flaxseed in baking—you can replace about one-quarter of the total amount of flour in the recipe with flaxseed and still get delicious results.

Solution #27

Pine Nuts

Have you had your phytonutrients today? Phytonutrients are offspring of the scientific marriage between natural foods and modern chemistry. Researchers have discovered that some foods *naturally* contain chemicals that may yield health benefits, and some of the chemicals are being isolated for medicinal purposes. For example, the cancer-fighting drug paclitaxel is derived from the bark of the Pacific yew tree, and lycopene (which may help prevent heart disease and cancer) comes from tomatoes. These chemicals, also called phytochemicals, are generally found in fruits and vegetables. Supporters of the organic movement believe that higher intake of fresh, minimally processed (even raw) plant foods is the key to reducing our risk of developing chronic diseases.

Pine nuts—the edible seeds of pines—are a newly recognized source of phytonutrients. Pine nut oil contains pinolenic acid, a fatty acid that stimulates the body to produce two natural appetite suppressants: the hormones cholecystokinin (CCK) and glucagon-like peptide-1 (GLP-1). Interestingly, there is a long history of people in Siberia munching on pine nuts or taking a tablespoon of pine nut oil to suppress their hunger when food becomes scarce.

Introducing pine nut oil into your diet is easy enough—a tablespoon of pine nuts contains only about 60 calories and makes an easy snack on its own, or it can be mixed into yogurt, cottage cheese, or pasta. Companies are also marketing pine nut oil in supplement form—capsules, chocolates, bars, and shakes to name a few—and according to their own research studies pine nut oil supplementation is associated with a drop of 7 to 10 percent in calorie consumption. Check out www.pinnothin.com for more ideas.

Solution #28

Enjoy 100-Calorie Snacks

Many of us really count on an afternoon snack to keep us going until dinner. But the problem with snacks—whether in the workplace, in the kitchen, or on the go—is that, most of the time, anything will do. You don't think as carefully about your snacking as you might about your next meal. Pass by vending machines and cinnamon buns. And because you do not plan for snacks, their impact on your diet can be difficult to assess. This can make it challenging to plan your regular meals.

One of the trickier aspects of snacking is that it's hard to pin down the right amount of food. Our perceptions of serving sizes or calories typically fail to match reality, and as a result we eat more than we need. Although our servings are strongly influenced by the sizes of our spoons, plates, bowls, and popcorn tubs, we can generally be satisfied by less food than we might expect. Enter the 100-calorie snack option. Limiting snacks to 100 calories makes it easier to plan regular meals, and you can snack away without worrying that you are going overboard.

Many food companies have taken this concept to the marketplace; you can now buy individually wrapped packages of cookies, candy, and other snacks that work within the 100-calorie framework. And it is easy to create your own 100-calorie snacks to save money and get more creative. But first you have to know what 100 calories look like. To get started, try the examples listed below. Put the portions into individual plastic bags at the beginning of the week, and enjoy them for your afternoon snacks.

20 mini-pretzels
5 chocolate kisses (try dark chocolate)
2 cups baby carrots
2 cups strawberries
All the celery you can eat

Research confirms that smaller portion sizes result in lower total daily calorie consumption. And once people become accustomed to the 100-calorie snack size, they are better able to regulate their portion sizes elsewhere. You'll find that 100-calorie snacks work well—as long as you eat just one!

Solution #29

Don't Overdose on Energy Bars

Energy bars appeared on the snack scene a few years ago in a blaze of misrepresentation. The secret that energy bar companies know (and now *you* know) is that the Food and Drug Administration allows manufacturers to label products as "energy" foods if they "contain calories." Makes you want to sit down with an energy pizza and an energy beer and forget about losing weight for a while. This "energy" label makes you think that you are getting something extra, when actually it's what trick-or-treaters have been enjoying for years. Sugar. Fat. Calories. All wrapped in shiny plastic.

Now before all you Mountain Dew–swilling, tire-swinging, rock-climbing X Games watchers drop your hacky sacks in a huff, let's get real. It is one thing if you have just scaled K2 and are looking for some quick calories and carbohydrates so that you can scramble down the scree before sundown to meet your yak train, but it's another if you are settling down for a quiet evening with your laptop and a chocolate chip peanut butter mint honey yogurt blast. The truth is that most people do not need extra carbohydrates even when they exercise—just because something might work for a high-intensity athlete doesn't mean that it's the best thing for you. And guess what? If carbs are all you're looking for, bagels work just as well. And while high-protein bars combined with exercise may be associated with increased muscle mass, protein can be consumed in lower-calorie forms too.

Ultimately, energy bars are repackaged, repurposed, and rebranded candy bars. Except that candy bars taste good. Stick with real food instead, and if you must open a wrapper, make sure to read the nutrition label before digging in.

Solution #30
Close the Kitchen After Dinner

Pick a time. It might be five-thirty if you eat earlier or have young children, or it might be later in the evening if you work long hours, have to juggle a spouse and a family, or live in Spain. Either way, choose a cutoff for your calories and commit to it. Snacking at night is one of the biggest challenges that dieters face, and it is often the last thing to go. People take solace in their evening cereal, scoop of ice cream, or, occasionally, beer. But there is a reason why many people successful at weight loss have closed down the kitchen and avoid nighttime snacks—it is because these calories *stick*.

Eating at night is associated with being overweight. While skipping meals is associated with a 30 percent increased risk of obesity, eating at night increases your risk by more than 50 percent! The timing of your food intake (affected by skipping meals, eating at night, and eating huge portions at limited meals), in addition to the calories themselves, impacts obesity risk.

This may have less to do with *what* you are eating than what you are doing *after* you eat. Meals throughout the day are usually preceded and followed by activity, which might be exercise but is typically the more mundane activity of daily life. Night eating is followed by . . . sleep. Because calories are not being burned as quickly, they may be more likely to be stored as fat. Studies have also shown that food eaten late at night is more likely to raise triglycerides, which are associated with metabolic syndrome and heart disease in addition to obesity.

Another concern is that your ability to regulate what you eat in a given day goes out the window if you are eating at night. For example, if you eat a high-calorie meal for lunch, you may be more inclined to eat less during dinner in order to compensate. But if the bulk of your snacking and consumption of high-fat treats occurs at night, it is likely that your overall daily calorie consumption will increase disproportionately. Whereas skipping breakfast makes you *over*compensate by eating too much throughout the day, cutting out nighttime snacks will likely result in an overall *reduction* in daily calories.

Other possible health benefits of eliminating nighttime snacking include less acid reflux, fewer asthma exacerbations, fewer trips to the bathroom, and better nighttime breath—not a health benefit per se, but your sleeping partner might appreciate it!

Solution #31

Sleep at Least Seven Hours a Night

There are not enough hours in a day. Despite our efforts to become more efficient, it seems as though we've made our days busier in the process. Smartphones mean that you have to check your messages. Hybrid cars give you an excuse to use your car to travel shorter distances. And the Roomba? Let's leave well enough alone.

In high school physics, we learned that a gas will expand to fill any container—it can fill a beaker or a swimming pool. Life seems like that sometimes. Your responsibilities, your daily list of things to do, your stress—they seem to expand to fill whatever time you have available. The end result? You have less free time than you thought you did. Twenty-first-century efficiencies somehow make room for more things to do, rather than give you more free time to do them.

But everybody sleeps. And most of us should sleep more. New data show that sleep affects our hormone balance in some interesting ways. The hormones ghrelin and leptin work in opposite ways to influence hunger and our sensation of being full. Ghrelin, produced in the gastrointestinal tract, tells your body to be hungry. Leptin, produced in fat cells, tells you to feel full. And these hunger/satiety hormones are impacted by your sleep habits.

If you are getting enough sleep at night, your leptin levels rise, and this results in your feeling full after eating less. But when you are not sleeping very much, ghrelin levels increase and leptin levels go down, and this makes you feel less satisfied. This has been well documented in people who sleep five hours a night as compared to eight hours a night. Their body weights also correlate with differences in sleep patterns. Obesity can be *three times more common* in night owls than in people who get a full night's sleep. Not only is poor sleep associated with obesity, but it is also predictive of diabetes, high blood pressure, and heart disease, not to mention depression and doing poorly in school. Some people suggest that poor diet and lack of exercise are not entirely to blame for the rapid rise in childhood obesity—maybe kids just aren't getting enough sleep.

Seven or eight hours appears to be the magic number. Start tonight.

3.
EVERY DAY

Every day you may make progress. Every step may
be fruitful. Yet there will stretch out before you an
ever-lengthening, ever-ascending, ever-improving
path. You know you will never get to the end of the
journey. But this, so far from discouraging, only
adds to the joy and glory of the climb.

— SIR WINSTON CHURCHILL

Two weeks go by quickly. And after fourteen days with the
Today Solutions, you are a little bit trimmer, a little bit more energetic, and a little bit more confident that you can really make
this work. And so the work begins.

Small changes are just that. They are discrete and incremental, but
they do require actual change. You are too smart to think that you can
lose weight by just tweaking the status quo. The trick is breaking down
those changes into small parts that you can easily understand and wrap
your mind around. Welcome to the Every Day Solutions.

It takes about twenty-one days to turn new behaviors into habits
that will stick with you. During the next three weeks, this comprehensive plan will help you retool your life—and lose ten pounds in
the process. The goal of these Every Day Solutions is to provide you
with many opportunities to impact your relationship with food and
activity in ways that work together and give you momentum. There

is a reason why they are called *Every Day* Solutions. Even though it should take you only three weeks to enjoy some substantial weight loss, this is just the beginning. Diet history teaches us that the most important predictor of success is *sticking with it*. If you go back to old habits and behaviors, the pounds will come back too. This means that it is time to start thinking about weight loss and wellness not as a destination, but as a journey. Once you get there, you want to stay there, and this means continuing to make good choices. It means always moving. *Every day*. The next three weeks are the beginning of your journey.

Any journey involves making choices along the way. In each of the categories described below, Solutions are separated into two groups: the first are Solutions that everyone should be able to follow; the second are Flex Solutions that you might be able to incorporate based upon your own lifestyle. The goal is to concentrate on the first group while experimenting with the Flex Solutions.

THE FIVE SENSES OF WELLNESS

Solutions are divided into five categories that break down a healthy lifestyle. I call them the five "senses" of wellness: Eat, Drink, Exercise, Act, and Live. Ideally, you should attempt to incorporate at least one Flex Solution from each category along the way.

Eat

These Solutions not only encompass nutritional advice and meal planning, but they emphasize some creative "life hacks" that you can use to alter your environment in subtle ways to ultimately reduce overall calorie intake. Solutions are organized by meal, because that is how we think about food. Look for specific action items around each meal as well as some meal ideas. Use the included recipes as learning opportunities instead of just following the directions.

Drink

You are already drinking six glasses of water a day. These Solutions are going to help you think more critically about other types of fluid intake—because calories are calories, no matter how you consume them. These Solutions are easy ways to make a change because it is so easy to substitute.

Exercise

While it is true that you can lose weight by just reducing your calorie intake, our greater goal is to improve health, and that does require exercise. However, the Exercise Solutions may be a little different from the aerobics class or jogging trail you are used to. This program incorporates your own body weight into a simple resistance training program to help build lean muscle, reduce belly fat, and increase metabolism so that you can more efficiently burn calories, even while you sleep. Add it to your warm-up or do it at your convenience at a different time of day.

Act

The main difference between exercise and activity is that exercise takes work and activity takes time. The Activity Solutions are all about finding more time and using it in better ways to get up and move. Walking thirty minutes a day, in whatever form, will help you lose weight and improve your fitness, even if you consider yourself fit already. The Solutions show you how to fit it in.

Live

In some ways, Lifestyle Solutions are the most fun to follow. Some of these Solutions might appear intuitive; others will surprise you. Did you know that shopping at Costco or getting your food without a certain additive can help you lose weight? How about using your iPhone or painting your dining room? These Solutions are fun to think about and easy to put into action. And like all the Solutions in this book, they are designed to help you lose a single pound. Maybe even more.

We have two goals here. The first is obviously to lose weight. But the second is to turn Solutions into habits, a program into a lifestyle, and a plan into the first three weeks of a very long journey. Where Every Day is Monday.

Hungry? Let's Eat.

THE EVERY DAY SOLUTIONS

Eat

32. Eat breakfast every day.
33. Eat eggs twice a week.
34. Avoid bagels.
35. Eat healthier bread.
36. Switch to a healthier breakfast cereal.
37. Use spreads sparingly.
38. Scoop or go halfsies.
39. Limit your menu.
40. Don't eat out of vending machines.
41. Hold the mayonnaise.
42. Substitute a vegetable for French fries.
43. Don't eat and drive.
44. Use microwave meals.
45. Limit eating out to two days a week.
46. Don't eat while watching television.
47. Eat at the table.
48. Eat a salad most days of the week.
49. Start with soup at least twice a week.
50. Eat fish at least once a week.
51. Eat tofu once a week.
52. Eat leaner red meat.
53. Do chicken right.
54. Eat beans at least once a week.

55. Limit carbohydrate servings to one cup.
56. Limit takeout or delivery to once a week.
57. Store the leftovers first.
58. Serve meals restaurant style, not family style.
59. Serve meals as courses.
60. Make vegetables your main course.
61. Sneak vegetables into other foods.
62. Don't eat your children's food.
63. Use less salad dressing.
64. Put out a vegetable platter.
65. Unload your baked potato.
66. Cut the fat.
67. Substitute quinoa for white rice.

Drink

68. Cut out sugar-sweetened beverages.
69. Avoid energy drinks.
70. Save your Starbucks.
71. Switch to skim.
72. Skip the diet soda.
73. Don't drink fruit juice.
74. Drink green tea.
75. Limit alcohol to weekends.

Exercise

76. Move slowly.
77. Push-ups.
78. The hands push.
79. The fly.
80. Good mornings.
81. The bent-over row.
82. Lateral raises.
83. Chair dips.
84. Chair extensions.
85. Curls.

86. Squats.
87. Split squats.
88. Calf raises.
89. Standing twists.
90. The Tibetan Twist.
91. The Superman/Banana.

Act

92. Climb stairs for ten minutes each weekday.
93. Walk during breaks at work.
94. Walk after dinner.
95. Walk your dog every day.
96. Walk before you shop.

Live

97. Make grocery shopping a healthier exercise.
98. Outsmart the supermarket.
99. Buy canned fruits and vegetables without additional ingredients.
100. Read food labels.
101. Don't eat from the restaurant breadbasket.
102. Ask questions in restaurants.
103. When you buy in bulk, store in servings.
104. Avoid all-you-can-eat restaurants.
105. Give drive-throughs the drive-by.
106. Share an entrée when you go out to eat.
107. Avoid MSG.
108. Make your Mexican food healthier.
109. Ask for a doggy bag when you order your meal.
110. Order a better pizza.
111. Think outside the bun.
112. Go grocery shopping without your kids.

EAT

Breakfast Solutions

Eat breakfast every day.
Eat eggs twice a week.
Avoid bagels.
Eat healthier bread.
Switch to a healthier breakfast
  cereal.
Use spreads sparingly.

FLEX Scoop or go halfsies.

SOLUTION #32
Eat Breakfast Every Day

The meal *is* the Solution.

But many people are still under the impression that breakfast means additional calories, and therefore additional weight. This is why many dieters make the mistake of skipping breakfast. Our moms always told us that eating a good breakfast is the best way to start the day, but more of us should have been listening. Only about half of American adults under age fifty-five eat breakfast every day, and most of us end up rushing the meal and making poor choices in the supermarket, drive-through, or coffee bar.

Eating breakfast is associated with a lower risk of obesity. This has been demonstrated in both men and women, in all age groups, and perhaps most poignantly in children. Some have hypothesized that skipping breakfast leads to consumption of more calorie-dense foods later in the day, resulting in higher calorie consumption overall. Breakfast skippers may snack more frequently and more impulsively, choosing high-carbohydrate foods that lead to weight gain. And eating fewer, larger meals each day may result in greater absorption of fat and sugar, for this reason, many diet programs recommend smaller, more frequent meals—including breakfast.

Research shows that just adding breakfast to your daily schedule can result in a weight loss of four pounds in a few months. And people who eat breakfast weigh an average of seven pounds less than people who wait until lunch to start eating. Try eggs, high-fiber cereals, and real fruit for starters, and try to limit your intake of sweetened cereals, white bread, and butter. Read on for more details.

Solution #33

Eat Eggs Twice a Week

A cardiologist recommending eggs? In a diet book?

Until recently, you could not find a physician who would allow an egg to get *near* one of his patients. Eggs typified a high-cholesterol, devil-may-care breakfasting lifestyle on the edge—and eggs would be the last thing you'd want to encourage in someone who had heart disease or wanted to avoid it. But as our understanding of nutrition has evolved over the years, it turns out that eggs are better for you than you (or your doctors) might think.

It all comes down to cholesterol. *Your* cholesterol levels. These numbers—the total cholesterol, LDL (low-density lipoprotein), HDL (high-density lipoprotein), and triglycerides—are important indicators of your overall risk of getting heart disease. We cardiologists work hard to make your numbers better with medication and lifestyle recommendations. Diet included.

So it would seem to make sense that if you eat foods high in cholesterol, your cholesterol levels should go up significantly. But it is not that straightforward. We now know that dietary cholesterol does not play that big a role in influencing your cholesterol levels—it is the saturated fats and especially the trans fats that you have to think about. While eggs are high in cholesterol, their saturated fat content is actually tolerable. Bottom line? Yes, you can still have eggs for breakfast. And you can knock out the saturated fat almost completely if you use egg whites rather than whole eggs. If you don't mind preservatives and a higher cost, packaged alternatives like Egg Beaters, AllWhites, and Better'n Eggs will also do the trick.

So eggs are safe. But do they help you lose weight? Absolutely. The low carbohydrate content of eggs makes them a great weight-loss food. They fill you up, and because they are low glycemic they help keep your blood sugar stable so you don't hanker for a muffin with your midmorning nonfat latte. Researchers have actually examined the impact of eating eggs for breakfast as compared to eating bagels, and they've found that eggs not only help you lose weight but also make you *feel fuller*. And the even better news? No significant differences in total cholesterol, LDL, or triglycerides. Could eggs be the perfect breakfast food?

Every Day Eggs

SIMPLE SCRAMBLE

What You Need

1 teaspoon olive oil
2 egg whites
Ground black pepper
Oregano (optional)

What You Do

Add oil to pan over medium heat.
Add egg whites and cook, stirring, until just set.
Season to taste.

What You Get

Calories 75 • Saturated fat 0.6 g • Cholesterol 0 mg
Sodium 110 mg • Fiber 0 g

SPINACH AND TOMATO SCRAMBLE

What You Need

1 teaspoon olive oil
1 sliced scallion
4 halved cherry tomatoes
½ cup chopped cooked spinach
2 egg whites
Ground black pepper or cayenne

What You Do

Add oil to pan over medium heat.
Add scallion and cook until transparent.
Add the remaining vegetables.
Add egg whites.
Cook, stirring, until just set.
Season to taste.

What You Get

Calories 113 • Saturated fat 0.7 g • Cholesterol 0 mg
Sodium 137 mg • Fiber 2.4 g

SALMON SCRAMBLE

What You **Need**
1 teaspoon olive oil
2 scallions, sliced
2 egg whites
1 ounce sliced smoked salmon
Ground black pepper

What You **Do**
Add oil to pan over medium heat.
Add scallions and cook until transparent.
Add egg whites and cook briefly.
Add salmon and cook, stirring, until just set.
Season to taste.

What You **Get**
Calories 116 • Saturated fat 0.9 g • Cholesterol 6.5 mg
Sodium 682 mg • Fiber 0.8 g

Solution #34
Avoid Bagels

A *New York Times* editorial once described bagels as "unsweetened doughnuts with rigor mortis." But they do taste good. They are actually one of my favorite foods, which makes it that much more difficult to present the following public Solution announcement:

Bagels are not great if you are on a diet.

A lot of people get fooled. Bagels are not fried, they aren't particularly sweet, and they do not seem like too much of a treat since they are not filled with chocolate chips or glazed. You might absentmindedly buy one the next time you are at your favorite coffee establishment, snack on one during an afternoon break, or just grab one from the bag in your office lunchroom on a Friday morning. But as with any food decision that becomes a habit, this one has consequences that add up—and quickly.

For many people, breakfasts or even snacks do not change much from day to day, so breaking the bagel habit is a good way to institute a small change in caloric intake for a great weight-loss result.

Bagels from a bakery or café usually have about 400 calories, and who can resist just a little cream cheese? At 100 to 150 additional calories per bagel, maybe we should try harder. With so many breakfast alternatives out there with fewer calories, fewer carbohydrates, and more nutritional value, a bagel with cream cheese should not be your first choice for breakfast, and it should be your last choice for a midmorning or afternoon snack.

A simple switch to an English muffin will satisfy your carbohydrate craving and with about one-third fewer calories than a bakery bagel. Add a little sugar-free jam or even a touch of vegetable oil spread and you will still take in substantially fewer calories. And if you must eat a bagel, consider buying frozen ones at the grocery store rather than buying from the bakery aisle; frozen bagels usually have about half the calories of fresh ones.

Solution #35

Eat Healthier Bread

Choosing whole-grain, high-fiber, and lower-calorie breads can help you lose weight. Whole grains fill you up more than bread made from refined flour, and given that fiber has no calories, eating high-fiber bread eliminates calories that you would otherwise take in, while still satisfying you. Studies show that people who eat white bread are hungrier two hours later and take in more calories at the next meal than people who eat whole-grain bread. This translates into real weight differences that you can sustain in the long term by continuing to eat bread that contains whole grains and fiber.

Other benefits include reducing insulin resistance and the risk of metabolic syndrome (more on that in chapter 5), preventing gallstones, and even lowering the risk of colon cancer. Whole grains are also associated with lower risks of heart failure, breast cancer, and diverticular disease. Not bad results for just making some different decisions in the bakery aisle.

But don't get fooled by misleading food labels. Buy only those breads with "whole wheat flour" as the *first* ingredient—"wheat flour" and "enriched bleached flour" can mean that some white flour is used. And don't be tricked by a healthy-sounding name—make sure you actually check the ingredients. The nutrition label should list the sodium and fiber content—look for less than 200 milligrams of sodium and at least

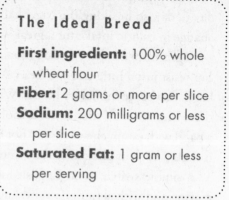

The Ideal Bread

First ingredient: 100% whole wheat flour

Fiber: 2 grams or more per slice

Sodium: 200 milligrams or less per slice

Saturated Fat: 1 gram or less per serving

two grams of fiber per slice. Finally, watch serving sizes. There is nothing worse than getting tricked by a cursory glance at the nutrition label only to find later that you have eaten double the calories to get what seems like the right amount of food.

Once you learn your way around the bakery section, it's easy to make the change. Just substitute whole wheat, high-fiber bread for white bread wherever you would normally eat sliced bread—at breakfast, or at any other time of day. It is not only healthier but it tastes heartier too. And if you have a family, buying better bread for them will start your kids (and maybe spouse) on a healthier course as well.

EVERY DAY BREADS	SOLUTIONS
Bagels	Thomas' Hearty Grains 100% Whole Wheat Bagels
Buns	Oroweat Whole Grain 100% Whole Wheat Hamburger Buns Oroweat Whole Grain 100% Whole Wheat Hotdog Buns
English muffins	Oroweat Whole Grain & Flax Oroweat 100% Whole Wheat
Pita pockets	Thomas' Sahara Pita Pockets Toufayan Multigrain Pita
Sliced bread	Milton's Whole Grain Plus Bread Nature's Pride 100% Whole Wheat Oroweat Country 100% Whole Wheat Oroweat Protein Health Sara Lee Hearty & Delicious 100% Multigrain

Solution #36

Switch to a Healthier Breakfast Cereal

If it has a cartoon character on the box, you should not be eating what is inside. Sugary breakfast cereals have been marketed to children for decades—if you think about it, it is one of the biggest advertising successes of our generation. Show kids a cartoon tiger or bumblebee eating something crunchy, and *POW!*—childhood obesity is through the roof. And even though you may not be entranced by cartoon characters or jingles, the sweet taste and the crunch appeal to the kid in you too.

The two things you should be looking for in a cold breakfast cereal are whole grains and fiber. Avoid refined grains because they will not fill you up and will leave you looking for doughnuts once you get to work. Avoid cereals with added sugar—if you can actually *see* the sugar crystals on the cereal, it is not a good sign. Choose cereals with fewer than 5 grams of sugar per serving, and if sugar is listed as the first ingredient, move on. And avoid trans fats (aka partially hydrogenated oils) and high-fructose corn syrup when possible. Remember, packaging is a form of advertising, so look at the nutrition label and ingredients for the real information. You may be surprised at some seemingly healthy choices that you actually should avoid.

CEREAL SOLUTIONS	CEREAL *NO*-LUTIONS
Fiber One Bran Cereal	Apple Jacks
Fiber One Honey Clusters	Basic Four
Kashi Heart to Heart Honey Toasted Oat Cereal	Cap'n Crunch
Post Grape-Nuts Trail Mix Crunch Cereal	Chex (Rice/Corn)
Quaker Oatmeal Squares	Cocoa anything
Raisin bran	Cookie Crisp
Shredded wheat	Corn Pops
	Crispix
	Froot Loops
	Frosted Flakes
	Honey Bunches of Oats
	Kix
	Product 19
	Rice Krispies
	Smacks
	Special K

Eating a healthy breakfast is not just about choosing the right cereal. It is also about choosing the right *amount* of cereal. As with chocolate, red wine, and pretty much anything else, the benefit is in moderation. A typical serving size is one cup. Fill the rest of your bowl with fruit and nonfat milk for a healthier breakfast.

Solution #37

Use Spreads Sparingly

Serving sizes are difficult to estimate when it comes to peanut butter, jelly, cream cheese, butter, and margarine. Using a tablespoon is messy and inconvenient. We use these spreads because they taste good, but it turns out that quantity does not play much of a role in how you enjoy your toast.

Try this experiment. Grab two halves of a bagel or two pieces of toast, and add your spread of choice—use it liberally on the first half or slice, and, on the second, spread it as thin as you can without being able to see through it. After you have eaten both, you may find that the first half was really almost too much; cream cheese, for example, was not meant to be applied like mortar.

Now consider the calorie savings. Two level tablespoons of peanut butter has almost 200 calories, and more fat than most hamburgers. And when was the last time you used only that much? Cream cheese, jelly, and buttery spreads are not quite as excessive, but cutting your serving size by half will add up significantly in a pretty short time. And also remember that the "individual serving" of cream cheese or peanut butter that you get at a coffee bar or café is not a mandate—spread judiciously and throw away the rest.

FLEX Solution #38
Scoop or Go Halfsies

While substituting English muffins or healthier bread for bagels is the most effective Solution, there are other options for those of us who don't want to make such a drastic change.

Consider the scoop.

The concept is simple. Use a fork or your fingers to scoop out the doughy interior of the bagel while maintaining the crust as well as the illusion. Scooping your bagel can reduce the number of calories by half. So eating two halves of a scooped bagel has the same calories as eating half a bagel, but it seems like you are eating more. Fooling your brain makes you feel fuller. For the typical oversized bakery bagel, this could mean upwards of 200 calories. But you do have to be careful that you don't make up in cream cheese calories what you lose in dough.

Before you get any crazy ideas, you should know that the "bagel scooper" has already been patented more than ten times, and inexpensive scoopers are available for purchase online if you don't like using conventional utensils at home. And if you buy your bagel at a bagel bakery or café? Have them do it for you. For two dollars, it is not too much to ask.

And remember, your knife can be used for more than just spreading cream cheese—use it to cut your bagel in half and cut some calories too.

Every Day Breakfast Solutions

OATMEAL

What You Need
1 packet plain instant oatmeal
1 tablespoon ground flaxseed
10 almonds
½ cup frozen blueberries
Cinnamon

What You Do
Following the directions
   on the package, add water
   to the oatmeal and microwave.
Add flaxseed, almonds, and
   frozen blueberries.
Add a dash of cinnamon.

What You Get
Calories 267 • Saturated fat 1.2 g • Cholesterol 0 mg
Sodium 77 mg • Fiber 9.2 g

BREAKFAST BURRITO

SERVES 2

What You Need
1 teaspoon olive oil
½ red pepper, diced
¼ yellow onion, diced
2 eggs plus 2 whites,
   beaten together
Ground black pepper
2 whole wheat tortillas

What You Do
Add olive oil to pan over
   medium-high heat.
Add vegetables and cook for
   three minutes.
Add eggs. Scramble until done.
Add pepper to taste.
Microwave tortillas for 30 seconds.
Wrap the eggs in the tortillas.

What You Get
Calories 254 • Saturated Fat 1.9 g • Cholesterol 212 mg
Sodium 518 mg • Fiber 4.8 g

PROTEIN SHAKE

What You Need
1 cup nonfat milk
1 tablespoon ground flaxseed
½ cup frozen blueberries
2 strawberries

What You Do
Mix in a blender.

What You Get
Calories 191 • Saturated fat 0.7 g • Cholesterol 4.9 mg
Sodium 132 mg • Fiber 6.0 g

CEREAL

What You Need
1 banana
1 cup cold breakfast cereal (see
    Solution #36)
½ cup nonfat milk

What You Do
Slice banana over cereal.
Add milk.

What You Get
Calories 271 • Saturated fat 0.7 g • Cholesterol 2.5 mg
Sodium 275 mg • Fiber 31 g

YOGURT PARFAIT

What You **Need**
½ cup sliced fresh strawberries
½ cup fresh blueberries
1 container (5.3 ounces) Oikos
   vanilla organic Greek yogurt
½ cup Kashi GoLean Crunch

What You **Do**
Put fruit in the bottom of a
   sundae bowl or a small dish
   or glass.
Add yogurt.
Sprinkle cereal on top.

What You **Get**
Calories 280 • Saturated fat 0 g • Cholesterol 0 mg
Sodium 112 mg • Fiber 7.9 g

Solution #39

Limit Your Menu

Many people think that they can make weight loss fun by introducing variety into their diets. There are thousands of recipes available for healthy meals, and it would seem that trying a lot of them would help you lose weight and keep food interesting at the same time.

But the data unfortunately suggest the opposite. Studies show that more food variety is associated with higher body weight. And more limited menus predict a greater reduction in fat and calorie intake as well as more weight loss. Exercise is different—adding variety to your exercise regimen through interval training, cross-training, and combining resistance training with aerobic workouts not only keeps exercise

Lunch Solutions

Limit your menu.
Don't eat out of vending machines.
Hold the mayonnaise.
Substitute a vegetable for French fries.

FLEX Don't eat and drive.
Use microwave meals.
Limit eating out to two days a week.

interesting, but it also introduces "muscle confusion" and improves long-term results. But lots of variety in your diet has the opposite effect—a high-variety diet stimulates your senses and therefore your appetite. The fewer choices you have, the less you will ultimately eat. Spend a few minutes watching the customers at a Las Vegas buffet and you will see what I mean.

Limiting your menu is a fairly novel concept in dieting, and it is not very popular, because it goes against the idea that we should eat for pleasure. You can still enjoy your meals, but by picking some staples that you can live with, you will eat more consistently. Less choice means fewer opportunities to make mistakes. Less choice means less spontaneity—which is honestly the last thing a dieter needs. Less choice means planning your meals in advance. Finally, less choice usually means limited portions.

Lunch is one of the easier meals in which to limit variety, because you tend to have a routine during the day at work or at home. Pick three to five lunches you like to bring from home or to eat out and rotate them throughout the week.

Solution #40
Don't Eat Out of Vending Machines

Vending machines have been around for over a hundred years, and today they provide everything from cigarettes to soda to hamburgers. But try to find something healthy to eat in a vending machine and you will more often than not come away empty-handed. Items in vending machines might be sitting there for long periods of time, so perishable items (like fruits and vegetables) are hard to find, particularly in the United States. Countries like Japan and the Netherlands do offer fresher and more substantial foods, but the foods are usually fried; it is hard to find a bag of mini-carrots among the croquettes and ramen noodles. Vending machines usually mean soda, chips, and candy bars in place of more balanced meals you could have brought more cheaply from home. Almost 5 percent of workers get their lunch from vending machines.

Don't be one of them. Hide your change, store your singles, and place a personal ban on vending machines.

Solution #41
Hold the Mayonnaise

Americans use it as a condiment on sandwiches. Europeans love it with French fries. Japanese incorporate it into sushi and salad. And Russians use it even more than ketchup. No matter where you live, mayonnaise is readily available, and it is also pretty simple to make with oil, egg yolks, and mustard, with lemon or vinegar added.

What this means from a nutritional standpoint is that one tablespoon has between 50 and 100 calories—and about 5 grams of fat. While most of the fats in mayonnaise are unsaturated, people generally use more than a tablespoon at a time. Holding the mayonnaise on your daily sandwich can drop 500 calories per week from your total intake. That is a pound in less than two months, just from changing your sandwich spread.

Miracle Whip is unfortunately not a great alternative. It actually has high-fructose corn syrup and sugar added to its "natural flavors," bringing you calories and fat similar to those in mayonnaise. Far from a miracle.

Fortunately there are some other condiments out there that are pretty good. Mustard is a great option. Although it can be high in sodium, mustard is generally used in smaller quantities than mayonnaise, and the result is fewer calories on your sandwich. Sweetened mustards are a bit higher in calories, but you can generally expect to consume about 90 percent fewer calories overall if you make the switch. Fat-free mayonnaise is another option, but it doesn't get many points in the taste department. Make your own tastier spread by mixing one and a half tablespoons of capers, one-third cup of fat-free sour cream, one teaspoon of garlic powder, and a dash of cayenne pepper in a food processor. It will taste fresher and you can make as much as you'll need for sandwiches or recipes.

Solution #42

Substitute a Vegetable for French Fries

It is estimated that the average American consumes about fifty-six pounds of frozen potatoes per year, mostly in the form of French fries. People who travel for work or who eat fast food frequently may eat at least three or four servings per *week*. Add some salt, ketchup, melted cheese, and gravy, or even (gulp!) mayonnaise, and you have taken the side dish to center stage, outdoing the rest of your meal in sodium, fat, and calories. Spuds are a universal staple—the United Nations declared 2008 to be the International Year of the Potato. So make this year the Year of the Substitute. Trade in your French fries for some healthy low-calorie, low-salt, no-fat steamed vegetables or salad, and trade in your old pants while you're at it. Substituting a steamed vegetable at lunch or dinner can save you upwards of 500 calories every time you would normally eat French fries.

FLEX Solutions

FLEX Solution #43

Don't Eat and Drive

Not only does eating while you drive divert your attention from more important things—like the road—but driving, in turn, diverts attention from what you are eating. It is rare enough to find good food choices on the road, whether you are eating at fast-food restaurants or buying snacks from gas stations or convenience stores. But eating while you drive makes bad choices even worse, because you lose your ability to calculate appropriate serving sizes. When a bag of chips or pretzels sits in the passenger seat, it is easy to munch absentmindedly. But if you take the time to sit down in a restaurant to have your lunch, you may actually decide against some of the fast-food outlets that would be more convenient if you are eating on the run. Convenience foods also tend to be high in carbohydrates and are often wrapped in plastic—you can't really eat a salad on the road. Better to avoid them.

FLEX Solution #44

Use Microwave Meals

Lunchtime is a challenging time of day, regardless of whether or not you are actively dieting. It is structured, yet unstructured—like recess for adults. You look over at one person and he's washing down pepperoni pizza with chocolate milk, and then you look at your own tired-looking peanut butter sandwich and wonder quietly about making a switch.

Enter the microwave meal. Seriously. Microwave meals have changed since the TV dinners you grew up with, or even the microwave meals you ate just five years ago. Responding to criticism about nutritional content, producers have worked hard to bring fat and sodium content down to real-world levels while maintaining some standards of good taste. True, the meals are processed food, but you could do worse.

Why are microwave meals a successful part of weight loss? It's simple math. Even when we are trying to limit our calories and be careful about portions, we are not all that accurate. In the same way that small plates are effective in limiting portion size, the predetermined small portions and limited calories of microwave meals are helpful too. Research shows that consistently using microwave meals as part of a diet results in weight loss over time.

Brands geared toward weight loss like Weight Watchers Smart Ones, Lean Cuisine, and Healthy Choice are a good place to start, but be aware that even among these better options there is a wide variety of fat, protein, and salt content. You need at least 300 calories to feel full, but make sure that the meal you buy has only "one serving," or else you could be inadvertently eating for two. To gain the greatest benefit, choose meals with fewer than 800 milligrams of sodium and more than 20 grams of protein—and the more fiber, the better. And if you are worried about filling up, throw in some frozen vegetables to bulk up your meal without bulking up yourself.

FLEX Solution #45

Limit Eating Out to Two Days a Week

This Solution is as easy as packing a brown paper bag. Studies show that over half of working Americans buy two or more of their weekday lunches rather than bring them from home. And overweight individuals are more likely to eat out. The most commonly cited reasons for buying lunch during the workday are based on misperceptions about convenience and cost, and the result is that people eat fast food. Fast food unfortunately accounts for almost half of lunches purchased during the workday. Even with expanded menus including apple slices and healthy salads, people more often turn to French fries and burgers, which supply too much salt and saturated fat, and too many calories. Add a soda, and you are easily looking at over 1,000 calories, with 75 percent of your salt intake for the day. For *lunch*.

There are real advantages to bringing your own lunch.

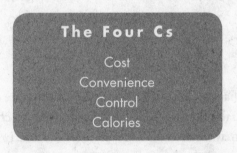

The Four Cs

Cost
Convenience
Control
Calories

1. **Cost savings.** When you buy food at the grocery store, you are in effect buying in bulk, which saves you money in the long run. When buying lunch, also consider the costs you do not even think about, like tipping in a restaurant, driving your car, and parking. They add up.

2. **Convenience.** You can pack some leftovers from last night's dinner, so all you need is a microwave. You can prepare the next day's lunch as part of your nighttime routine, or just incorporate doing it into getting the kids off to school or packing your bag for the day.

3. **Control over your portions.** When you bring your own lunch, the food you bring is the food you eat. It doesn't allow for a last-minute decision to order appetizers or dessert, and it does not require willpower. What's in the bag is all you get, and the portions you serve yourself tend to be much more reasonable than the ones you pick out from a drive-through menu when you are starving.

4. **Calories.** When you make your own lunch, you control the amount of spread on your sandwich and dressing on your salad (both of which are used in excess in restaurants). And unless you have a deep fryer in your office, you can really eliminate trans fats entirely by bringing lunch from home. If you typically eat a fast-food lunch five days a week, this change could mean a difference of 2,500 calories in just one week.

But you still have to make good choices. Concentrate on whole-grain breads and low-salt and low-fat deli meats, and use no cheese if you can help it. Avoid mayonnaise in favor of mustard and bring low-calorie dressing for your salads. Load up on carrots, green pepper slices, and jicama—anything with a healthy crunch. Pack fruit instead of cookies for dessert.

Every Day Lunch Solutions

PB & BANANA SANDWICH

MINI-CARROTS • CELERY STICKS • YOGURT

What You Need

2 tablespoons low-fat peanut butter
1 medium banana, sliced
2 slices whole wheat bread
½ cup minicarrots
2 celery sticks
1 container nonfat yogurt

What You Do

To make the sandwich, spread peanut butter and place banana slices on bread.

What You Get

Calories 707 • Saturated fat 4.1 g • Cholesterol 5.0 mg
Sodium 745 mg • Fiber 14.2 g

QUESADILLA

SALSA • GREEN/RED PEPPER SLICES • APPLE

What You Need

2 six-inch flour tortillas
¼ cup shredded part-skim mozzarella
½ red pepper, sliced
½ green pepper, sliced
2 tablespoons salsa
1 apple

What You Do

To make the quesadilla, place cheese, vegetables, and salsa between the tortillas and microwave for 30 seconds.

What You Get

Calories 440 • Saturated fat 4.2 g • Cholesterol 16.4 mg
Sodium 582 mg • Fiber 10.4 g

TURKEY WRAP

MINI-CARROTS • APPLE SLICES WITH PEANUT BUTTER

What You **Need**

2 slices turkey breast
2 tablespoons hummus
1 whole wheat pita bread
½ cup mini-carrots
1 apple
2 tablespoons low-fat
   peanut butter

What You **Do**

Make sandwich with turkey and
   hummus inside the pita.
Slice apple and spread with
   peanut butter.

What You **Get**

Calories 557 • Saturated fat 3.5 g • Cholesterol 18.3 mg
Sodium 1,170 mg • Fiber 13.1 g

TUNA SALAD

CRACKERS • GRAPES • YOGURT

What You **Need**

1 can (3 ounces) light tuna in water
1 celery stalk, chopped
¼ cup shredded carrots
1 small box raisins
4 whole wheat crackers
1 cup grapes
1 container (6 ounces) nonfat yogurt

What You **Do**

To make the salad, combine
   tuna, chopped celery,
   carrots, and raisins.

What You **Get**

Calories 427 • Saturated fat 0.9 g • Cholesterol 45 mg
Sodium 637 mg • Fiber 6.5 g

CHEDDAR AND APPLE SANDWICH

VEGETABLE SOUP

What You Need
½ apple, sliced thin
1 slice cheddar cheese
2 slices whole wheat bread
1 cup canned vegetable soup

What You Do
To make the sandwich, place apple and cheese slices on the bread.

What You **Get**
Calories 492 • Saturated fat 7.1 g • Cholesterol 34.5 mg
Sodium 962 mg • Fiber 8.9 g

Solution #46

Don't Eat While Watching Television

You have heard this before—probably when you were in junior high school and wanted to put on your favorite show while the dinner table was being set (that's what we did). For some people, dinner is family time, and television is forever a point of contention between kids and their parents. For those who live alone or who are empty nesters, television provides an easy distraction while we eat. And for those who work from home, it seems like the television is always on, particularly when we eat. In fact, about 40 percent of Americans watch television during dinner every night.

But research indicates that the more television we watch, the greater our risk of becoming overweight. This correlation has been recognized in children and adolescents as well as adults. The reasons may include advertisements for high-calorie snacks, less leisure-time physical activity, and eating mindlessly while we watch television.

Multiple studies indicate that we eat more—in some cases between 35 percent and 70 percent more—if we are watching television at the same time. One study found that watching television while eating a meal was associated with consuming over 200 extra calories. And the type of calories we consume while watching may also make a difference. We tend to snack on high-carbohydrate and high-salt foods while in front of the television. And when we are distracted from how much we are eating, we eat more. The studies that examine the effect of eating while watching television focus on mealtimes, but the larger effect may actually occur later at night. So if the television is on, keep your mouth closed—and if you're eating, turn off the television.

Solution #47

Eat at the Table

If you eat while walking, standing at the refrigerator, or hunched over the kitchen counter, you will not enjoy your food as much and won't feel as full. Part of the enjoyment of food is the actual experience of eating. Sit at the table, even if you are eating alone. Make an event out of your meal. Have a designated eating space in your home or apartment—avoid the sofa, coffee table, or computer desk. Pay attention to your food, and eat deliberately. Be mindful of

Dinner Solutions

Don't eat while watching television.
Eat at the table.
Eat a salad most days of the week.
Start with soup at least twice a week.
Eat fish at least once a week.
Eat tofu once a week.
Eat leaner red meat.
Do chicken right.
Eat beans at least once a week.
Limit carbohydrate servings to one cup.

FLEX Limit takeout or delivery to once a week.
Store the leftovers first.
Serve meals restaurant style, not family style.
Serve meals as courses.
Make vegetables your main course.
Sneak vegetables into other foods.
Don't eat your children's food.
Use less salad dressing.
Put out a vegetable platter.
Unload your baked potato.
Cut the fat.
Substitute quinoa for white rice.

what you are eating, and take the time to enjoy it now, so that you will not be hungry later.

Solution #48
Eat a Salad Most Days of the Week

Salad has two big advantages for people trying to lose weight. The first is that people typically eat salad at the beginning of a meal, when they are hungrier. The second is that salads are generally low in carbohydrates and fat and are low energy density, so you fill up on fewer calories. The more salad that you eat, the fewer calories you will consume overall. One study found that eating a large salad before a meal reduced the total number of calories by 12 percent. If you have a sweet tooth, try eating salad at the end of your meal. It will fill you up and you will be less likely to have dessert.

1. **Go green.** The more greens in your salad, the more likely it is to fill you up with fewer calories.

2. **Think bright and dark.** Colorful vegetables and darker-colored greens offer more nutrients with fewer calories. Many people choose iceberg lettuce because it is the lettuce they grew up with. It also tends to be a bit cheaper than other varieties. But at only about 1 gram of fiber per cup, it is not the best option if you are trying to boost your fiber intake. Spinach and romaine lettuce have double the fiber, at only about 10 extra calories per cup.

3. **Add fruit.** Adding fruit to your salad will make it taste great and reduce the need for high-calorie dressing.

4. **Avoid meats and cheeses.** This is a salad, not a sandwich—the best weight-loss salads are made without meat or cheese. If you feel the need, make sure you use grilled rather than

fried meat, and use cheese as a garnish rather than as a base ingredient.

5. **Use a healthier dressing.** People often justify using a creamy, high-fat dressing because they feel entitled to it—they *are* eating salad, after all! Unfortunately, many of these dressings get most of their calories from fat. Buying fat-free or low-calorie dressings and requesting them in restaurants can reduce your calorie and fat intake by about 80 percent with little effort. Many people use vinegar and oil because they believe it is a healthier option, but fat-free and low-calorie dressings are better weight-loss choices. If you eat a salad every day, you will probably cut out 1,000 calories a week.

DRESSING (1 tablespoon)	TYPE	CALORIES	CALORIES FROM FAT
Caesar	Regular	78	76
	Low cal	17	6
French	Regular	73	65
	Fat free	21	0
Italian	Regular	43	38
	Fat free	7	1
Ranch	Regular	70	68
	Fat free	17	1
Russian	Regular	74	69
	Low cal	23	6
Thousand Island	Regular	59	50
	Fat free	21	2
Vinegar and oil	Regular	72	72

Solution #49

Start with Soup at Least Twice a Week

Eating soup every day is associated with good health and weight loss. I am not talking about cream of potato, cheesy broccoli, or French onion soup with a gooey layer of melted Gruyère on top. Healthy soups are broth-based, low in salt, and high in vegetables. Homemade soups are probably the best option—and you save a lot of money too by making a pot on Sunday and having servings available throughout the week.

So why soup? This gets into an interesting weight-loss concept—volumetrics. Whereas *energy density* refers to the number of calories per unit of food weight, *volumetrics* is the idea that foods larger in size take up more space in your stomach. They make you feel fuller and also satiate you psychologically. So if you combine energy density and volumetrics, soup is an obvious Solution. The high water content creates a large volume of food with relatively low energy density, and it really does fill you up. This has ramifications for weight loss.

Research supports eating soup as part of a weight-loss plan and suggests that it may be even more effective than drinking extra water with your meal. Eating a bowl of soup before a meal has been shown to result in consuming 20 percent fewer calories overall. Look for soups low in calories—a high-fat, high-calorie cream-based soup or cheesy soup would be a step in the wrong direction. Although they do fill you up, high-fat soups fill you up with calories too. That's the wrong kind of volume.

SOUP SOLUTION

SERVES 4

What You **Need**

4 cups diced tomatoes
2 carrots
2 celery stalks
½ onion
1 zucchini
1 cup green beans
2 cloves garlic
4 cups vegetable broth
Basil
Oregano
Pepper

What You **Do**

Chop the carrots, celery, onion, zucchini, green beans, and garlic.

Combine all the ingredients in a pot and bring to a simmer over low heat.

Simmer for 1 hour.

Season to taste.

What You **Get**

Calories 92 • Saturated fat 0.1 g • Cholesterol 0 mg
Sodium 1,000 mg • Fiber 5.1 g

Solution #50

Eat Fish at Least Once a Week

Fish is a great heart-healthy addition to any diet. The American Heart Association recommends at least one serving per week, primarily for its cardiovascular benefits—it improves cholesterol levels, may lower blood pressure, and reduces the risk of cardiac events like heart attacks.

But if that doesn't move you toward the seafood aisle, maybe *this* will: eating fish is associated with losing weight. We are not taking about breaded, fried, or fast-food fish that comes served as a "-wich," has an "O" after the filet, or arrives in a basket with a side of curly fries and hush puppies. Enjoy fresh fish pan seared, broiled, grilled, or sushi style to get the benefits without the batter. Studies show that lean fish (like cod) and fatty fish (like salmon) *both* help with weight loss. Fish is expensive, so don't forget that canned tuna works to reduce weight too.

As with many dieting strategies, it is not just about what are you doing, but also about what you are *no longer* doing. If you are eating fish (cooked in a healthy way), you are not eating red meat, and you are not eating fried chicken. And you are probably not eating fast food.

Solution #51
Eat Tofu Once a Week

Tofu has been enjoyed by vegetarians and vegans for decades as an excellent protein source that is low in fat, and these same qualities make it a great weight-loss food. Derived from soy milk, tofu really does not have that much flavor. Its blandness makes it an ideal Solution for use in many different types of dishes, and it can be incorporated into any meal of the day. It is naturally low in calories. Also, soy protein may be beneficial in lowering your cholesterol. Studies show that substituting tofu for other protein sources is associated with reduced body fat—but eating it as a supplement to your meaty meal will not necessarily help you lose weight.

So the best way to incorporate tofu into your diet is by eating it instead of another protein source that might be higher in fat, like red meat or cheese. But you can also use it as a meat "extender"—it will increase your portion size without adding significantly to the calories. There are a few approaches to using tofu in cooking; you can make it the centerpiece of the dish, or just sneak it in there to provide some protein and make you feel fuller. Because it does not have much flavor on its own, it is easy to do either.

But first you have to buy it—many Westerners find the tofu refrigerator aisle pretty intimidating, but it doesn't have to be. Tofu comes in many textures, from "extra firm" to "silken," and several in between. The firmer varieties hold their shape on the grill or in the wok, and they work very well as red meat substitutes in barbecues or stir-frys. To get the best results, make sure you buy the right kind for the recipe you are following. Softer versions crumble easily and work as substitutes for scrambled eggs, ricotta, or even cream cheese in some recipes. Varieties on the silken end of the spectrum can substitute for mayonnaise or sour cream, with significantly less fat, and can thicken soups or sauces.

You can even have tofu for breakfast—the high protein content will help keep you full during the morning and less likely to reach for an unhealthy snack. This recipe for a five-minute tofu scramble serves two people and contains fewer than 250 calories per serving. Enjoy anytime.

TOFU SCRAMBLE

SERVES 2

What You Need
1 teaspoon olive oil
½ onion, chopped
½ green pepper, chopped
2 scallions, chopped
16 ounces firm tofu, crumbled
Soy sauce
Turmeric
Black pepper

What You Do
Heat oil.
Add onion, green pepper, and scallions and sauté for 2 minutes.
Add tofu and sauté for 2 minutes.
Add soy sauce, turmeric, and pepper to taste.
Cook for 1 minute.

What You Get
Calories 231 • Saturated fat 3.2 g • Cholesterol 0 mg
Sodium 185 mg • Fiber 6.7 g

Solution #52

Eat Leaner Red Meat

Many people who are trying to lose weight figure that they will have to eliminate red meat from their diet. And while there are benefits to reducing your consumption of red meat, you can also enjoy it as part of a weight-loss program. The key is buying the leanest type of beef that you can. Hamburger beef that is 90 percent lean will only be about 50 calories per ounce, whereas beef that is 75 percent lean will be about 80 calories per ounce. The difference in the calories provided by fat is amazing, and those calories can add up quickly.

Different *cuts* of beef have very different fat and calorie content. For example, top sirloin is one of the leanest cuts, and rib eye is one of the fattiest. In restaurants, hamburgers tend to be made from fattier meat; the fat makes them juicier and easier to cook. And if you want to order a steak in a restaurant, it is important to choose wisely. Steak is one of the few dishes for which the restaurant tells you specifically how much food you are about to eat. If you choose the nine-ounce filet mignon, you will be getting essentially half the fat and calories of the sixteen-ounce T-bone.

CUT OF BEEF (100 g or 3.5 ounces)	CALORIES	SODIUM (mg)	CHOLESTEROL (mg)	SATURATED FAT (g)
Top sirloin	172	58	68	2.2
Tenderloin	207	68	78	3.2
Strip loin	209	58	71	3.3
Flank	236	61	71	4.3
Rib eye	248	54	69	5.7
T-bone	247	71	70	5.3

Also keep in mind that how you prepare your steak or burger at home will help determine the amount of fat that reaches your plate. Pan-frying meat allows the meat to soak up its own fat, which makes it juicier but also higher in calories and fat. Broiling or barbecuing it allows the fat to drain away, George Foreman style.

Some dieters try to bypass these issues by substituting turkey for red meat. Turkey can be a better choice, but that is not always the case. The table below shows the estimated calorie and fat content of a four-ounce serving of four different burgers: ground beef, lean ground beef, regular ground turkey, and lean ground turkey breast. Can you guess which is which?

GUESS THE MEAT!	CALORIES	FAT (g)
A	210	13
B	200	11
C	170	8
D	160	7

Not so confident now? It turns out that most preparations of lean ground beef (C) at less than 7 percent fat, have about the same number of calories and grams of fat as lean ground turkey breast (D). Regular ground turkey (B) has a slight advantage over regular ground beef (A). But the striking thing is that lean ground beef is a better choice than regular ground turkey, which may include some dark meat and skin, which amps up its calorie and fat content.

When you buy deli meat, pay attention to added salt and sugar as well as to fat content. There are healthier options out there, like Applegate Farms Organic Oven-Roasted Turkey Breast and Turkey Bacon, which are very low in saturated fat and sodium. The bottom line is to buy lean, and substitute lean turkey for beef when you can. Not only will you consume fewer calories, but you may reduce your risk of colon cancer and other health problems that some studies have linked to high beef consumption.

Solution #53

Do Chicken Right

Not all chicken is created equal. And given that Americans eat about fifty pounds of chicken per year (that means several times per week), there are a lot of opportunities to make things better.

First, many people do not recognize that chicken varies in its fat and calorie content according to the cut. Chicken breasts are the lowest-calorie part of the chicken to eat, with dark meat and wings at the opposite end of the scale. Choose breasts rather than thighs or legs in the supermarket and look for "all-white-meat" on the packages.

Next, remove the skin. Removing the skin can cut the fat in a serving of chicken by 50 percent. To put things into perspective, removing the skin from a roasted chicken breast takes off about 40 calories, more than 4 grams of fat, and more than a gram of saturated fat. Although cooking the chicken with the skin on will keep the meat from drying out and make it tastier as well as juicier, it may also prevent any sauces, rubs, or marinades you use from penetrating the meat. There is also the possibility that some of the fat from the skin will "melt" onto the meat. I recommend removing the skin *before* you cook.

Finally, the preparation. Once you admit to yourself that "nuggets," "fingers," or anything shaped like a dinosaur is not a style of cooking, you are on to something. Simmering chicken in a stew or roasting it are the healthiest ways to prepare it, while stir-frying and deep-frying result in a much higher-fat meal. Many people stir-fry as a way to incorporate vegetables and meat together in the same dish, but keep in mind that oil is fat, which means extra calories—even if you use olive oil. One trick is to bake the boneless strips or pieces of chicken first, and then add them to the wok to mix with vegetables and sauces just before serving. Following these steps can make chicken a healthy high-protein, low-fat staple of your diet.

Solution #54

Eat Beans at Least Once a Week

While not as sexy as acai berry or as exotic as Korean pine nuts, beans and other legumes are versatile and diet-friendly, and they also contain phytochemicals that enhance your health. Beans are one of the few foods that are actually enjoyable at breakfast, lunch, and dinner. Split a breakfast plate between black beans, scrambled egg whites, and micro-waved mixed frozen vegetables and you will feel full all day. Try pinto beans at lunch, with some chicken or lean beef, veggies, and spicy salsa. Dinner can be lentils, your choice of meat, and steamed vegetables. Beans are incredibly high in fiber (one cup gives you half of a day's recommended intake), and the fiber teams up with high water content to satisfy you.

Some people avoid beans because of their relatively high calorie content. True, if you are counting calorie for calorie, beans contain similar calories to meat. But because meat has no fiber, eating beans will fill you up and have you take in fewer calories overall. One study found that people who ate beans weighed seven pounds less than those who didn't.

While Americans are not accustomed to eating beans frequently, many cultures have created entire cuisines around them. While doing research in Costa Rica during medical school, I enjoyed *gallo pinto* (a mixture of black beans and rice) for breakfast every day, and had black beans as a side dish with nearly every meal. Five years later I was a medical volunteer in Nepal, and I ate *dal bhat* (lentils and rice) twice a day. Each cuisine offered delicious, satisfying dishes and did not leave me craving more familiar ones. Bean immersion is not for everyone, but if you find a few types you enjoy and can prepare easily, try incorporating them into a meal at least once a week. If you are buying canned beans, purchase only vegetarian beans (bacon tends to ruin the benefit!). Try these ideas for starters.

Bean Solutions

GALLO PINTO

What You Need

2 teaspoons olive oil
1 onion, finely chopped
2 cloves garlic,
   finely chopped
1 red pepper,
   finely chopped
1 cup cooked black beans
1 cup cooked white rice
Fresh cilantro
Black pepper

What You Do

Heat olive oil.
Add onion, garlic, and red
   pepper and sauté for 5
   minutes.
Add black beans.
Add rice and simmer.
Add cilantro and black pepper
   just before removing pan
   from the heat.

What You Get

Calories 649 • Saturated fat 1.7 g • Cholesterol 0 mg
Sodium 9.8 mg • Fiber 19.3 g

DAL BHAT

What You **Need**

10 tablespoons lentils
Chili pepper
Fresh ginger, minced
1 onion, finely chopped
Fresh garlic
2 tomatoes, chopped
Fresh coriander leaves,
    chopped
1 cup cooked white rice

What You **Do**

Boil lentils with 5 cups of
    water, until soft, about 30
    minutes.
Mash lentils and add chili and
    ginger to taste.
Sauté onion, garlic, and toma-
    toes separately.
Once the onion and garlic are
    browned, add them with the
    tomatoes to the lentils.
Add a handful of coriander.
Serve with rice.

What You **Get**

Calories 521 • Saturated fat 0.4 g • Cholesterol 0 mg
Sodium 229 mg • Fiber 15.9 g

Solution #55

Limit Carbohydrate Servings to One Cup

Portion control is a key component of a healthy and sustainable weight-loss program, because manipulating *how much* we eat can be as important as choosing *what* we eat. One food group in which we often misjudge amounts is carbohydrates.

Don't worry. We are not about to go on an anti-carb tirade here. The Flex Diet does not discourage you from eating pizza, pasta, bread, or rice—or even dessert sometimes. But what is amazing is just how much we can eat without realizing it. Carbohydrates can be tricky because it is easy to consume large amounts without recognizing the caloric impact. Research has shown that we tend to overestimate what a portion size should be for high-carbohydrate foods, as compared to high-fat foods, and that, unfortunately, our portion sizes tend to correlate with our body mass index. That is to say, the bigger we are, the more we eat.

Creating a moratorium on carbohydrates may help you lose weight, but it's just not that much fun. Every burger wants a bun. But if we learn more about how to regulate portion sizes, we may be better able to continue enjoying the foods we prefer while still gaining some benefit from smaller servings, and therefore fewer calories.

Grab a measuring cup from your kitchen drawer and use it. With cereal. With rice. With pasta. Eat the same meal you were planning on, but with just one level cup of the carbohydrate. One cup of cooked pasta or rice contains about 200 calories, and one cup of cold *nongranola* breakfast cereal typically has between 100 and 150. Most of us serve ourselves at least double these amounts, partly because we use large plates and bowls, and partly because we have a tough time eyeballing the portions without a little bit of help. If you are one of the 30 percent of people who eat cold cereal for breakfast, you could drop 500 calories a week by measuring out a cup before putting it in your bowl. Subtract another 100 or more calories per spaghetti dinner or Chinese take-out meal. One cup is all it takes.

FLEX Solutions

FLEX Solution #56
Limit Takeout or Delivery to Once a Week

Unless you live in New York, take-out and delivery options are pretty much limited to pizza and Chinese food. And here's the real tip: both are heavy hitters—very high in carbohydrates, fat, and salt. If there are any vegetables, they are typically drowning in oil or melted cheese. Sure, they taste great, but try to limit takeout or delivery to once a week—this includes weekends. The food you prepare at home will be healthier, and you will avoid the split-second decision making on the telephone that sometimes prompts you to make the less healthy choice at the last moment.

FLEX Solution #57
Store the Leftovers First

People typically cook way too much food. Most cookbooks provide recipes for a minimum of four people, and often eight. For many people who live alone or have small children, it can be difficult to cook a meal or even order out without ending up with extra food. Add in our difficulties with estimating appropriate portions of pasta and rice (somehow we rarely have the same problem with broccoli), and you end up with a full pot or casserole dish with more servings than mouths to feed.

How do *you* deal with this situation? Until now, you might have served yourself seconds, and then stolen a bite here and there as you put things away or cleaned the dishes. Solution? Put away the leftovers *first,* and freeze them so they are not as accessible. This will limit your portion to the one on your plate. If you can, store extra servings individually, so you know how much food you will need to take for lunch or dinner the following day without getting into the same situation. If you are cooking for a family, have your spouse or an older child put away the extra food as you serve. Cutting recipes in half is a helpful idea as well—recipes in this book are geared toward one or two servings to take some of the guesswork out of it.

FLEX Solution #58

Serve Meals Restaurant Style, Not Family Style

It is hard enough to get everyone around the dinner table at the same time, whether you live with roommates, a significant other, or family. In an effort to streamline the process of doling out food, many people put the casserole dish or serving bowl in the middle of the table or just serve themselves directly from the wok or pasta strainer. While eating out at restaurants is not without its problems, one benefit is that you do not typically get more than one serving of each food (although the serving itself may be too large). But at home, you have free reign until the food is gone. By leaving pots and pans on the kitchen counter or range, where they belong, you can separate cooking from eating. Serve each person's food on a plate, and keep the casserole dish away from the table. If you have a dining room, use it. Even the few steps separating you from the kitchen will help to keep you from going back for seconds.

FLEX Solution #59

Serve Meals as Courses

When you eat a nice meal at a restaurant, there are often several courses—you might get soup or a salad, followed by your entrée. And even when you are planning to get something sweet at the end of the meal, you sometimes decide that you do not really want it anymore by the time your server comes around. This is less likely when you are at home. Even if you do eat salad, for example, you may tend to put everything on one plate or bring it all out at the same time. And if your food is presented to you all at once, you will tend to eat it more quickly and finish more of it. Your stomach does not have enough time to signal to your brain that you are full until it is too late. Instead, you can pace yourself by serving your meal as different courses. Put salad or soup on the table first. And consider dividing your main course—start with the vegetable, and then bring out the meat and starch. And don't eat dessert until you have put all the other dishes away.

FLEX Solution #60

Make Vegetables Your Main Course

What would go well with broccoli tonight?

Not a question you typically ask yourself as you make a stop at the market on the way home or go through your refrigerator to get dinner ready. Typically, we center our meals around a meat—usually beef or chicken—or sometimes a starch, like pasta. Take a look at the dinner plates of families at home across America, or at meals served in restaurants, and you will usually find a common proportioning of meat, starch, and vegetables. The meat takes up half the plate, the starch takes up at least a quarter, and vegetables (if they make it to the plate) might take up the final quarter. And we usually eat what we are served. These skewed proportions direct us to eat more meat and saturated fat and less fiber.

So plan your dinners differently. Think first about what vegetables you are going to eat for dinner. Then fill half your plate with vegetables and arrange your meat and starch around them. If you make the meat and starch more of an afterthought, you will end up eating less of them. Researchers have found that people will eat more vegetables and take in fewer calories overall if meals are presented this way. And the same studies find that people are not any hungrier after eating more vegetables as compared to a higher-calorie meal with more meat.

You can prepare larger portions of your usual broccoli, or peas and carrots, or you can experiment with new recipes for a vegetarian main dish. There are lots of great possibilities at websites like www.allrecipes .com and www.theveggietable.com. And here are a few easy ideas to get you started.

Vegetarian Solutions

GRILLED VEGETABLE KEBABS

EAT THREE

What You Need
3 cherry tomatoes
1 cup sliced zucchini
1 cup sliced green pepper
6 mushrooms
1 onion, cut into 1-inch pieces
1 tablespoon olive oil
Black pepper

What You Do
Put cherry tomatoes, zucchini, green pepper sticks, mushrooms, and onion onto skewers, brush with olive oil, and add black pepper to taste.
Grill until the vegetables are tender and have a seared edge.

What You Get
Calories 208 • Saturated fat 1.9 g • Cholesterol 0 mg
Sodium 10.5 mg • Fiber 5.5 g

ASPARAGUS WITH ALMONDS

What You Need
10 asparagus spears
Olive oil cooking spray
Lemon juice
½ cup sliced roasted almonds
1 cup brown rice

What You Do
Sauté asparagus over high heat with some cooking spray, and then add a splash of lemon juice. Add some sliced almonds and serve with brown rice.

What You Get
Calories 531 • Saturated fat 2.2 g • Cholesterol 0 mg
Sodium 5.7 mg • Fiber 12.5 g

VEGETABLE PITA POCKETS

EAT TWO

What You Need
¼ cup chopped tomato
¼ cup chopped cucumber
¼ cup chopped red onion
¼ cup crumbled feta cheese
Oregano
Black pepper
1 whole wheat pita

What You Do
For the filling, mix chopped vegetables with a tablespoon of feta cheese. Season to taste.
Warm filling in the microwave for 30 seconds and serve in the pita pocket.

What You Get
Calories 297 • Saturated fat 5.9 g • Cholesterol 33 mg
Sodium 765 mg • Fiber 6.2 g

FLEX Solution #61

Sneak Vegetables into Other Foods

Parents have been trying to get their kids to eat vegetables since the beginning of time. The most recent concept is to avoid the usual confrontation between your toddler and a plate of brussels sprouts in favor of hiding vegetables in other foods like mashed potatoes, tomato sauce, muffins, or even ground beef. But whether or not you have kids, you can still sneak some vegetables into your own food.

Rather than make things complicated by having to think about how many shredded carrots you are going to bake into a chocolate cake, start simply by incorporating purée vegetables into other foods. Steam vegetables until they are soft, and then purée them in a blender. Cauliflower and zucchini purée works great in creamy sauces like Alfredo, and it also adds some substance to your macaroni and cheese. You can use broccoli and spinach as a green addition to your pasta sauce, lasagna, or casserole, reducing the need for too much cheese or meat. Make a blender's worth of puréed vegetables on Sunday and use it up by the end of the week—you will get more servings of vegetables and take in less fat and fewer calories.

FLEX Solution #62
Don't Eat Your Children's Food

After you finish your own meal, you glance out of the corner of your eye at your four-year-old's pizza, fish sticks, or grilled cheese sandwich, and while he is looking the other way . . . you pounce. He wasn't going to eat it anyway, right? Sometimes you're being sneaky, and sometimes it's an absentminded bite as you put away dishes, pack some crackers for a long drive, or fix an after-nap snack. And at a restaurant? Those chicken fingers are *not* going to waste.

Surveys suggest that one in five moms finishes her children's meals for them, and one in four will eat some of her kids' food in an attempt to get them to eat more. This can easily add up to 1,500 extra calories in just one week when you consider all the fries, nuggets, and crackers children eat—and this is in addition to the normal "adult" meals and snacks. These calories often go unnoticed, and most people don't count them in their internal food diary—they are not planned and are often hard to quantify. Just a handful of goldfish crackers or a pretzel here and there does not seem like much, but your waistline isn't so picky.

Let's face it, kids' food tastes good. It is salty, high in carbohydrates, and often deep-fried. (There is little chance that you are stealing steamed lima beans from your children's plates.) Even if *you* order the salmon and vegetables, you can quickly ruin your healthy choice by adding a garnish of fries and half a cheeseburger. One obvious solution is to give your kids healthier food—so if you do steal some it will not have as much of an impact. Even so, their calories shouldn't become yours.

FLEX Solution #63

Use Less Salad Dressing

Determining the appropriate portion size of commercial salad dressing can also be a challenge. While the bottle might list calories and grams of fat per tablespoon, most people use much more than this. Using an actual tablespoon is cumbersome enough at home, but in a restaurant the dressing has often been added beforehand, complicating the issue. Whether you are eating out or at home, have your salad dressing on the side. Dip your fork into the dressing and then use it to grab some salad. This way you are guaranteed to get some dressing on every bite, while at the same time limiting your serving size significantly. You can expect to decrease the amount of dressing you use by about two-thirds, and you will find it easy, convenient, and actually less messy than eating salad the conventional way.

FLEX Solution #64

Put Out a Vegetable Platter

The interval after school or work and before dinner is a dangerous time for dieters. You are tired and hungry and perhaps a little less patient, and as a result you may make poor choices with snacks before sitting down for your evening meal. Anticipate this by having a ready supply of vegetables that you like to snack on. Red and green peppers, celery, carrots, and even broccoli are low-energy-density foods that will curb your hunger without adding many calories. If you have a tough time eating raw vegetables, have low-calorie dip on hand to add some flavor. Guiltless Gourmet makes delicious black bean dips, and you can make your own dip by mixing nonfat yogurt with lemon juice, thyme, oregano, parsley, and pepper. But be careful how much you use, or else the appetizer will become the meal.

FLEX Solution #65

Unload Your Baked Potato

Remember a few years ago when the baked potato became a popular diet food? The idea was to avoid French fries or onion rings in restaurants by providing a "healthier" option. But as with many things, we find a way to get around the healthier possibilities—in this case, by adding bacon, cheese, and sour cream.

The good news is that baked potatoes are back. And some small changes can turn them into Solutions for you. A baked potato with healthy toppings can actually be your main course—add some cooked ground turkey, corn, black beans, and salsa and you no longer need rice or fried taco shells. Or add chopped tomato and onion and a little bit of feta and you have a more substantial salad. Use cottage cheese, or even a little bit of applesauce, instead of sour cream. Baked sweet potatoes are an even better option; they are higher in fiber and protein and will keep you fuller than a similar serving of rice or even pasta.

FLEX Solution #66

Cut the Fat

Did you know that paper towels are a weight-loss tool? While many people are accustomed to using paper towels or napkins to soak up the little pools of oil that surface on pizza, the same strategy can be helpful with a variety of foods. Placing cooked meat on paper towels for thirty seconds on each side before serving will get rid of excess fat. This might not seem like a significant intervention, but research shows that you can remove 2 grams of fat (nearly *20 calories*) from a hamburger by doing this. Another trick when preparing ground beef for tacos or chili is to briefly rinse the cooked meat under hot tap water and then put it back in the skillet or pot for the rest of the cooking process. Rinsing a serving of ground beef has been shown to reduce the fat content by about 6 grams, or about *60 calories*. You can still use paper napkins when you eat out, but if you pour your water over your burger, it probably will not go over very well.

FLEX Solution #67
Substitute Quinoa for White Rice

White rice is a staple in many people's diets, and this makes it an ideal target for a Solution. True, rice is a complex carbohydrate, which means it takes longer to digest than simple carbohydrates like those in pastries or sweets. However, white rice is a refined starch, so it has a high glycemic index and isn't a very good weight-loss food. Consider substituting quinoa as a high-protein, high-fiber alternative to rice. While many people assume that quinoa is a grain, it is actually more similar to spinach, chard, or beets. But it will fool you. When you boil it in water or prepare it in a rice cooker, it takes on a texture much like white rice or even couscous.

One cup of cooked quinoa has about 40 fewer calories than the same amount of white rice, but the real benefit is in the carbohydrates. White rice has almost 15 times more grams of carbohydrate than quinoa, and quinoa gives you 5 more grams of fiber and double the protein. The bottom line is that quinoa will not only help you cut calories but will fill you up so that you end up eating less. For some fast results, try substituting quinoa everywhere you would normally use rice. Another great solution is to use brown rice instead of white rice—it is a naturally low glycemic index carbohydrate that will satisfy your appetite and help you control your portion sizes.

Every Day Dinner Solutions

REFRIED BEANS

TORTILLAS • TORTILLA SOUP

What You Need

1 cup pinto beans
½ cup canned tomatoes
½ teaspoon chili powder
¼ teaspoon cumin
¼ teaspoon oregano
¼ teaspoon cayenne pepper
¼ teaspoon salt
¼ cup water
1 teaspoon lime juice
2 whole wheat tortillas
1 cup prepared tortilla soup

What You Do

To make the refried beans, combine beans, tomatoes, seasonings, water, and lime juice in a saucepan.

Cook over medium heat until soft.

Mash.

Microwave tortillas for thirty seconds.

Serve the beans with the tortillas and soup.

What You Get

Calories 595 • Saturated fat 0.7 g • Cholesterol 0 mg
Sodium 1,490 mg • Fiber 34.8 g

PASTA WITH VEGETABLES

SERVES TWO

What You **Need**

Olive oil cooking spray
2 cups sliced mushrooms
½ cup sliced green onions
1 cup chopped tomatoes
1 package frozen spinach, defrosted
    and drained
2 cups cooked whole-grain pasta
¼ cup feta cheese

What You **Do**

Spray a pan with cooking spray.
Sautée mushrooms and onions.
Add tomatoes and spinach and
    cook until heated through.
Pour over the pasta.
Garnish with feta cheese.

What You **Get**

Calories 322 • Saturated fat 3.0 g • Cholesterol 17 mg
Sodium 571 mg • Fiber 12.5 g

ORANGE VEGETABLE STIR-FRY

What You **Need**

2 tablespoons soy sauce
2 tablespoons corn starch
Olive oil cooking spray
Garlic, minced, to taste
1 cup diced onions
1 cup green pepper strips
1 cup broccoli florets
½ cup orange juice
Black pepper, to taste
1 cup cooked rice

What You **Do**

For the sauce, combine soy sauce and
    corn starch with 1 cup of water.
Coat a saucepan with cooking spray
    and heat to hot.
Add garlic and sauté.
Continue cooking as you add onions,
    green pepper strips, and broccoli.
Add the sauce.
Add orange juice and black pepper.
Serve over rice.

What You **Get**

Calories 916 • Saturated fat 0.3 g • Cholesterol 0 mg
Sodium 946 mg • Fiber 9.1 g

TURKEY BURGERS AND FRIES

SERVES TWO

What You *Need*
Black pepper
1 egg white
½ pound lean ground turkey breast
2 cups frozen sweet potato fries
1 cup frozen corn
2 whole-grain buns
Green salad

What You *Do*
Preheat oven to 450°F.
To make the burgers, mix
    pepper and egg white with
    ground turkey and shape
    into 2 patties.
Place the burger on foil and
    bake for 30 minutes.
Bake fries at same time.
Microwave corn.
Place the burgers on the buns
    and serve with salad.

What You *Get*
Calories 600 • Saturated fat 4.0 g • Cholesterol 80 mg
Sodium 696 mg • Fiber 8.7 g

MAKE-YOUR-OWN PIZZA

What You *Need*
4 tablespoons tomato sauce
1 multigrain English muffin, cut in
    half and toasted
1 cup shredded part-skim mozzarella
Seasonings (such as oregano,
    red pepper flakes, or prepared
    Italian seasoning)

What You *Do*
Spread the sauce over the
    muffin halves.
Sprinkle mozzarella on top.
Toast until crisp.
Season to taste.

What You *Get*
Calories 467 • Saturated fat 11.8 g • Cholesterol 66 mg
Sodium 1,250 mg • Fiber 3.0 g

DRINK

Solution #68

Cut Out Sugar-Sweetened Beverages

Call them soft drinks or soda, tonic or pop, fizzy drinks or diabetes in a can. Sugar-sweetened beverages, or SSBs, as they are referred to in scientific circles, are high in calories and low in nutrition, and they add inches to your waistline—if you let them.

Previously, soft drinks were sweetened with sugar or corn syrup, but modern soft drinks are often flavored with high-fructose corn syrup. High-fructose corn syrup is panned by nutritionists and physicians because it has been linked to obesity and diabetes. The high calorie content and low nutritional value of soft drinks are unfortunately eclipsed by the drinks' convenience; high consumption, particularly among kids, is the result. It is estimated that soft drinks contribute around 8 percent of our total calorie intake, and about 63 percent of us drink them regularly, despite the increased availability of no-calorie options.

Soft drinks are scientifically proven to be associated with obesity. It has been estimated that drinking just one can of soda a day could correspond to a weight gain of about a pound a month. One study demonstrated that decreasing soft drink consumption by 82 percent corresponded to over four pounds of weight loss.

One of the challenges that soft drinks present is a confusing message regarding portion size. For canned beverages, this is not an issue, but many people would be surprised to read the label on many apparently single-serving-sized bottles of soda to find that they are intended for two separate servings—usually clocking in at least 250 calories apiece. Drink one of these bottles daily for just two weeks and you will have consumed a pound's worth of calories without much else to show for it.

But remember, the ideal alternative to sugary soda is . . . no soda at all. If you are swearing off soda, the best choice is to drink a low- or no-calorie beverage without an artificial sweetener—try water. If you need a little kick of flavor, try one of the new brands of "enhanced" water, but make sure that it has no calories, and ideally no artificial sweeteners. Ayala's Herbal Water uses only herbs like mint, lemongrass, and ginger to create an organic, zero-calorie, and zero-preservative option that is gaining popularity.

Solution #69
Avoid Energy Drinks

"Energy" drinks were once an accompaniment to vodka enjoyed exclusively by celebrity tweens, but they now constitute a fifth food group relied upon by shift workers, high school students, and even medical trainees trying to look cool. Energy drinks are a fixture of extreme sports and college campuses; many energy junkies enjoy several each day, and more on the weekend.

Energy drinks are quickly reshaping the whole "sugar-sweetened beverage" landscape into a taurine and guanine-infested jungle of high calories and even higher caffeine content. The potential health risks of energy drinks are for another discussion, but isn't it enough to know that they have been outlawed in several European countries?

Like any sugar-sweetened beverage, energy drinks are generally high in calories, and multiple "servings" are often packaged within the same can or bottle. A unique feature of energy drinks is how frequently they are consumed together with alcohol to fight its depressive effects so that the user can stay up later and party like a rock star. By keeping you awake, this combination can result in higher alcohol intake overall, which means more calories from alcoholic beverages in addition to worse cognitive impairment, more microwave burritos at the convenience store (see "worse cognitive impairment"), and a wicked hangover the following morning. Rock star, indeed.

If you must use "energy"-laden products, consider lower-calorie options like 5-hour Energy, Red Bull (smaller serving as compared to other drinks), or even old-fashioned black coffee. And get some sleep.

Solution #70

Save Your Starbucks

Starbucks is everywhere. And many people sit on those purple faux-velvet sofas on a daily basis, often without recognizing the ramifications of their purchases. The difference between a Grande and a Venti seems vague when you are face to face with the barista. And when whipped cream is offered for free, few people want to pass it up. Whereas New York City passed a law requiring that nutritional information be posted for chain restaurants, most of us do not know what we are drinking. Check out the nutritional information from the Starbucks website for these Grande-sized drinks.

STARBUCKS GRANDE-SIZED DRINKS

DRINK	CALORIES	SATURATED FAT (g)	SUGARS (g)
Coffee (black)	5	0.0	0
Caffè Americano	15	0.0	0
Caffè Latte (nonfat)	130	0.0	18
Caffè Latte (2%)	190	4.5	17
Caffè Latte (whole)	220	7.0	16
Caffè Mocha (2%)	260	4.0	31
Coffee Frappuccino Light Blended Coffee	130	0.0	16
Coffee Frappuccino	240	2.0	40

DRINK	CALORIES	SATURATED FAT (g)	SUGARS (g)
Java Chip Frappuccino Light Blended Coffee	200	3.0	24
Java Chip Frappuccino Blended Coffee	340	5.0	52
Hot Chocolate (2%) without whipped cream	300	4.5	39
White Hot Chocolate (2%) with whipped cream	490	13.0	62

To put the issue into nutritional perspective, it helps to know that the American Heart Association recommends that you take in less than 7 percent of your daily calories from saturated fat. If you take in 2,000 calories daily, that's just 140 calories from saturated fat. At about 9 calories per gram, that's 16 grams of saturated fat a day. Or about two large whole-milk lattes.

Changing your latte from whole milk to nonfat is an easy 90-calorie Solution, and it translates into 3,500 calories (one pound) in just over five weeks. Going from a Java Chip Frappuccino to the lighter version saves you 140 calories—or one pound in just twenty-five days. Swear off the White Hot Chocolate entirely and you have just lopped off almost 3,500 calories *in one week*.

If you are a stickler for your favorite drink, then just go smaller. The difference between a small and a large 2% latte is 90 calories, and the difference between a small and a large 2% mocha is 140 calories. Coffee Frappuccino? 160 calories. White Hot Chocolate? 210. That's a pound in seventeen days.

Oh, and by the way . . . a large White Chocolate Mocha (whole) with whipped cream has similar calories and saturated fat to a McDonald's Quarter Pounder with Cheese. Seems like if you cut out a beverage like that, every day, you would not only be saving toward your retirement, but you might have a better chance of reaching it at a healthy weight.

Solution #71

Switch to Skim

The average American consumes almost two cups of dairy products daily, including milk and milk products, like cheese. And while this represents an increase over the past thirty years, we are still not quite up to the two to three cups a day that are recommended. We are also consuming more low-fat and no-fat dairy products than ever before. Whole-milk consumption has fallen by 70 percent, and lower-fat choices have more than doubled. Mozzarella cheese (with less fat than Swiss or cheddar) is now America's favorite.

That's the good news. However, many of us still consume 1% or 2% milk rather than nonfat. Keep in mind that "whole" milk only has about 3.25% to 3.5% fat content, so slimming down to 2% doesn't impact your calorie intake significantly. Nonfat milk tastes better now than it did when you were a kid, thanks to the addition of a small amount of dietary fiber that makes the milk look and taste more like 2%, but without the calories.

Type of Milk (1 cup)	Calories
Nonfat	90
1%	105
2%	125
Whole (3.25–3.5%)	150

Even if you do not have a glass of milk with breakfast or lunch, think about all the places where milk or milk products slip into your calorie intake, from breakfast cereal to coffee drinks, to shredded cheese on your salad, pasta, or Mexican food. Take a cue from Solution #70—you could decrease your daily intake by 100 calories by making the switch from whole to skim, and by as many as 35 calories for just coming down a notch from 2% to skim. If this seems like too much to ask, then consider combining half whole milk and half reduced-fat or skim for a few weeks to transition. It is a painless way to drop calories and still enjoy what you normally eat and drink.

Got Solution?

FLEX Solutions

FLEX Solution #72
Skip the Diet Soda

Many people automatically assume that choosing "diet" foods is a good way to lose weight. At least that is what the commercials suggest. Taking in fewer calories would seem to be the obvious way to shed pounds—so bring on the diet soda, diet candy, diet pound cake, and diet pudding!

But there is some bad news for you diet cola addicts out there: drinking diet soda (and using sugar substitutes in general) is *not* associated with weight loss. In fact, one study found that a daily can of diet soda was associated with a *41 percent increased risk* of becoming obese—actually higher than the risk for drinking a comparable amount of regular soda. Body mass index has been shown to increase by 1.5 points in those who drink three diet sodas daily.

Is anything in dieting easy?

Research on artificial sweeteners has yielded some interesting findings that teach us a lot about how our bodies respond to food. Studies demonstrate that substituting artificial sweeteners in foods like yogurt leads to increased consumption of calories overall—and weight gain—during just two weeks. And not only has diet soda been associated with weight gain, but one study even points toward an increased risk of metabolic syndrome and diabetes among diet soda drinkers. Why would this be?

Sugar-loaded foods are obviously high in calories; this is one of the reasons why dieters try to avoid them. But when you consume sugar substitutes, a few things happen. Subconsciously, you believe that you are making a good choice by *not* having a sugar-sweetened drink, and so you simultaneously make other choices (like the cheeseburgers and fries on your tray) that might not be so helpful. And although you may enjoy the faux sweet taste of the sugar substitute, your body is not so easily fooled. When the diet soda doesn't deliver, your body makes you crave the real thing.

When you eat sugar, your body responds by increasing insulin levels. But in the absence of real sugar, the insulin levels may spike anyway, causing hypoglycemia (low blood sugar). Guess how your body deals with that? You crave more sugar! Try to avoid choosing between regular and diet soda. We know that regular soda promotes weight gain. And the concept here is that the choice may be easier than you think. You don't have to drink either one.

How sweet it was.

FLEX Solution #73
Don't Drink Fruit Juice

A general rule for weight loss is to avoid consuming liquid calories. This applies mostly to sugar-sweetened beverages like soda and energy drinks, but fruit juice cannot be ignored. While juice certainly has some nutritional benefit, it is also relatively high in calories, and unlike the actual fruit, it does not really fill you up.

Research shows that many people who drink juice regularly are overweight. This is because, with regard to calories, your body does not differentiate between juice and a candy bar. Both are high in simple sugars. Also, people don't tend to "count" liquid calories as part of their overall intake, so they tend not to compensate by limiting calories in other areas. But one cup of orange juice or unsweetened apple juice contains about 120 calories, so you might be consuming a pound's worth of calories each month if you have orange juice every day with breakfast.

If you must have your juice, aim for the juice, the whole juice, and nothing but the juice. Many products, especially those aimed at kids, masquerade as juice but go by names like "punch," "blend," or even "cocktail," and they are often sweetened with sugar. Grabbing a glass of fruit "drink" with your morning bagel gives you the same number of calories as a cheeseburger. For breakfast.

If you substitute the fruit itself for the fruit juice, you will consume about half the calories. The high water content and fiber in the fruit also fill you up, and may actually reduce your appetite for the rest of your meal or for snacks throughout the day. The easiest Solution is to drink something else.

FLEX Solution #74
Drink Green Tea

Americans consume significantly less tea than coffee, but Chinese and Japanese people have been drinking a lot of tea, including green tea, for years. High consumption of tea is now being examined as a factor in the lower prevalence of some cancers in East Asians, as well as differences in body type between East Asians and Westerners.

Catechins—antioxidant compounds also found in chocolate and wine—are what seem to provide the health benefits in tea. There are studies that suggest that green tea can prevent cancer, reduce heart disease, delay aging, and do pretty much everything you might like a beverage to do. And green tea can also help you lose weight.

Multiple research studies have found that drinking green tea instead of other beverages with the same caffeine content can result in weight loss of several pounds over just a couple of months. But you may need to drink more tea each day than the amount of coffee you normally drink in order to achieve a weight-loss effect. The majority of studies used about four cups a day.

Another benefit of drinking green tea rather than coffee is that you will probably consume less sugar and cream (or nondairy creamer) as well.

FLEX Solution #75
Limit Alcohol to Weekends

Cardiologists appreciate the benefits of modest alcohol consumption. You may already know that drinking alcohol in moderation (one drink a day for women, and one or two drinks a day for men) is associated with a lower risk of heart disease. Alcohol has antioxidant and anti-inflammatory effects, and multiple research studies have found that people who drink alcohol have a lower likelihood of developing coronary artery disease or having heart attacks.

But the problem with alcohol for people trying to lose weight is that alcoholic beverages tend to provide calories without much nutritional benefit. A martini every day after work or a glass of wine with dinner will provide you with at least 500 calories each week. And many people enjoy larger servings, even within one glass. This adds up before you know it. Take a look at the calories contained in each of these commonly enjoyed drinks and do the math for your own cocktail.

Beverage	Calories
Light beer (12 oz.)	100
Gin, Rum, vodka, or whiskey (one shot)	100
Wine (red/white) (5 oz.)	100
Martini	120
Bloody Mary	120
Cosmopolitan	130
Beer (12 oz.)	150
Gin and tonic	200
Screwdriver	200
Mai tai	300
Piña colada	300
Margarita	330
Rum and Coke	350
Dessert wine	350
Mudslide	800

It is difficult to estimate how the health benefits of a daily drink stack up against the risks associated with being overweight. To significantly reduce your overall liquid calorie intake, meet yourself halfway and limit your alcohol consumption to weekends.

EXERCISE

This easy-to-follow exercise program requires only *three hours* of your time during the next three weeks. The goal is to use resistance training to increase your lean muscle mass, raise your metabolism, and reduce belly fat and drop weight. You will start by using your own weight as resistance. In the future you could also invest in a set of dumbbells.

Why have resistance training in a weight-loss program? Many cardiologists recommend aerobic exercise like running or tennis, and I agree that these are great options. In fact, the Flex Diet incorporates more cardiovascular exercises in the Activity Solutions as well as throughout the *Your Way* Solutions. But many exercise physiologists would also argue that resistance training is the key to maintaining a healthy weight and a fit body.

Any weight-loss program should include diet modification through portion control, eating breakfast every day, and avoiding late-night snacks. But as we limit our calories and lose weight, about 25 percent of the loss is in the form of muscle. At the same time, fat is slowly replacing muscle mass as we grow older. Thus people appear to become fatter over time, even if their weight remains the same.

The Solution is to add resistance training to your weight-loss plan. The advantage of resistance training is that you may increase your resting metabolic rate by as much as 15 percent. An extra pound of lean muscle on your frame can translate into your burning an extra 50 calories per day. A more muscular body will burn more calories at rest, even while you are watching television or sleeping.

Packing on some muscle will make you look better too. Remember, muscle is more dense than fat, which means that a more muscular person could weigh the same or even a bit more but appear thinner than a less muscular person. Another way of thinking about it is to note that fat takes up more space than muscle. Using your own body for resistance or experimenting with light weights will make you more toned and lean. These exercises are designed to avoid making you bulky. Instead, they will help you drop a dress size or pants size, and the calories you will burn will help you lose weight overall. This effect has been documented in research studies that found that people lost weight by lifting weights, even though they were consuming an extra 400 calories per day.

There are five major muscle groups that we are going to work out: chest, back, arms, legs, and core. Remember that spending additional time on a "problem area" will not burn more fat in that specific region—you can build muscle in a targeted area, but fat burning is more of a generalized process that occurs everywhere. Follow the directions closely with respect to how much time to spend on each exercise, and give yourself thirty seconds between each set before moving on to the next one. As with any exercise program, it is advisable to clear it with your own doctor before getting started.

Solution #77

Push-ups

These are already included in your Warm-Up Solution (see Solution #12), and now we

---

FLEX Solution #76

Move Slowly

While resistance training and lifting weights are great for fitness and weight loss, many people are not exercising to their best advantage. *Move slowly.* Exercise science shows that taking longer to do the same resistance exercise improves your fitness, builds more muscle, and burns more calories. As you go through the Exercise Solutions, move purposefully and try not to rush through the exercises to get them done. The actual time spent is part of the benefit. These exercises have specific recommendations regarding the number of repetitions as well as the number of seconds that you should hold each pose. This strategy, despite taking longer, helps you build muscle faster. More efficient exercise means decreasing your overall exercise time. That is why you only need to do these exercises for one half hour, twice a week.

---

will add some more. Lying on your stomach, put your hands at shoulder width on the floor. Now place your toes on the floor and maintain a straight back as you straighten your arms. Keep your chin up. Now bend your arms at the elbow until your chest almost touches the floor. Push with your hands until your arms are fully extended again. Some people will find this difficult, and will want to do easier push-ups with their knees on the floor. But an even better option is to keep you feet on the floor (and your knees off of it) and place your hands on a sofa, a table, or even a wall. The goal is to keep your back completely straight and isolate the muscles you are working on. Count three seconds on the way up, three on the way down. Start with a goal of ten for one set. Do two sets.

Solution #78

The Hands Push

Stand with your feet at shoulder width. Put your palms together in front of you. Have your fingers pointed upward and your elbows at shoulder level. For a count of five seconds, press your palms together as hard as you can. Then relax for three seconds. Do ten repetitions.

FLEX Solution #79

The Fly

For an additional chest exercise, try this one using dumbbells. Start by lying on a bench or other hard surface with your arms at your sides and your hands grasping the dumbbells. Extend your hands upward, elbows pointed outward and arms straight. Slowly lower the dumbbells to your sides while keeping your arms slightly flexed and your elbows pointed outward and toward the floor. Extend your arms so that your elbows are at the same level as your shoulders. Now bring the dumbbells together in a hugging motion until they touch gently. Five seconds down. Five seconds up. No rest in between. Do five repetitions.

Solution #80

Good Mornings

This is a variation of a weight-lifting exercise that uses just the weight of your arms. Stand with your feet at shoulder width and your arms at your sides. Raise your arms to the horizontal position at shoulder height. Now slowly bend at the waist, keeping your back straight and looking straight forward, until your back is horizontal like a table. Then slowly return to an upright position, keeping your back straight and looking forward. Keep your knees slightly bent and your abdominal muscles tensed the entire time. Five seconds down. Five seconds up. Do ten repetitions.

FLEX Solution #81

The Bent-over Row

For additional back work, kneel over a bench or sturdy chair, by placing your right knee and hand on it for support. Grasp the dumbbell in your left hand with your arm extended. Lift the dumbbell close to your side, bending your elbow and bringing your upper arm to the horizontal. Slowly extend your arm again. Five seconds up. Five seconds down. Do ten repetitions.

Solution #82

Lateral Raises

Stand with feet at shoulder width with your arms at your sides. Raise your arms to the horizontal over five seconds and then hold this position for five seconds. Lower them over five seconds. Do ten repetitions.

Solution #83

Chair Dips

Sit on a sturdy, stable chair and grasp the sides of the seat close to your buttocks. Straighten your legs, keeping your heels on the floor, and push your body gently off the chair so that you are supported by your flexed arms. Lower your body slowly until your arms are bent at a ninety-degree angle. Then slowly straighten your arms to return yourself to the starting position. Three seconds down, three seconds up. Do ten repetitions.

Solution #84

Chair Extensions

Now sit on the chair in an upright position—your back should not be resting against the chair. Extend your left arm in front of you and rest your right arm at your side. Lower your left arm slowly as your raise your right arm to the extended position. The rhythm should be fluid, as if you were walking. The key with this exercise is to do it slowly—take five seconds to switch arm positions. Do ten repetitions.

FLEX Solution #85

Curls

To further tone your arms, stand with your feet at shoulder width and your arms down, your palms facing forward, holding dumbbells at your sides. Slowly bend your arms, keeping your elbows at your sides—they will have a tendency to flare outward. The weights should be in front of you the entire time. Five seconds up, five seconds down, ten repetitions. Do two sets.

Solution #86

Squats

Stand with your feet close together. While keeping your back straight and looking forward, bend your knees slowly until they are flexed at a ninety-degree angle. Then slowly rise to standing. Five seconds up, five seconds down, ten repetitions.

Solution #87

Split Squats

Stand with your feet at shoulder width. Step far back with one of your legs. Keep your arms straight in front of you. Lower your body slowly until your back knee almost touches the floor. Keep your back straight and your head up. Now slowly rise to standing. Alternate your legs. Three seconds up, three seconds down, five repetitions on each leg.

Solution #88

Calf Raises

To further strengthen your legs, stand with your feet at shoulder width, toes pointed forward. Slowly rise to your tiptoes and then slowly return your heels to the floor for a count of twenty. Then do twenty repetitions as fast as you can safely. Do two additional sets of this exercise, the first with your toes pointed inward, and the next with your toes pointed outward.

Solution #89

Standing Twists

Stand upright with your feet at shoulder width. Clasp your hands behind your head and extend your elbows backward so that they are aligned with your shoulders. Now slowly turn your torso to one side as far as you can go without moving your hips—take five seconds to make the turn. Hold your position for five seconds and then twist the other way. Keep your head facing forward in line with your torso, and keep your abdominal muscles flexed the entire time. Do ten on each side.

Solution #90

The Tibetan Twist

Stand upright with your arms crossed over your chest. Your fingertips should be on your shoulders. Now extend your arms to the sides, keeping them horizontal at shoulder height. Your palms should be facing downward. Spin your torso slowly from side to side as in the standing twist, holding your position at each side before you twist the other way. Do five on each side and then return to the starting position. Repeat once more.

Solution #91

The Superman/Banana

For the final core exercise, lie on the floor on your stomach. Extend your arms straight ahead and look forward as though you were flying (Superman). Now slowly lift your hands and head as you lift your feet off the floor. You should keep your arms and legs straight so that you are bending slightly at your waist. Hold this position for ten seconds. Then quickly flip onto your back, keeping your head off the floor, your arms extended over your head, and your feet raised a few inches off the floor. Keep your arms and legs straight so that you are bent slightly at the waist (Banana). Hold for ten seconds. Alternate positions every ten seconds until you have done this exercise for a minute. Repeat once more.

ACT

Solution #92

Climb Stairs for Ten Minutes Each Weekday

Do you take an elevator every day?

If you have an elevator at work, you probably take it up and down at least four times a day, instead of taking the stairs. If you go to the mall, the doctor's office, or just about anywhere, you have the option of taking the elevator or escalator, or, again, just taking the stairs.

When you ask most people why they do not take the stairs more often, it is usually not a question of motivation but rather one of time. People generally believe that climbing one flight of stairs takes more time than taking the elevator to the second floor. But an enterprising group of university students has presented data showing that it actually takes about twice the amount of time to take the elevator one flight up or down as compared to walking the stairs. Walking to the third floor is probably the break-even point for time spent.

So if you are not saving time by taking the elevator or escalator, then why not just take the stairs? The authors of more than fifty published studies have looked into this, and they have found that simple behavior patterns keep sending us toward the elevator. It's not even a matter of being lazy. We just don't think about it all that much.

It's time for us to become more mindful. Signs are effective reminders, but they aren't used in many places. And unless you buy multiple copies of this book and place them strategically in front of elevators and escalators all over the country (hmmm . . .), you are stuck with this Solution: climbing stairs for ten minutes each workday.

We do know that climbing stairs burns calories. Various studies have tried to determine how many, but the number changes depending on your body weight and how fast you are moving. For the sake of argument, let's go with an estimate of 0.15 calories per step up, and 0.05 calories per step down. Others have estimated 10 calories per minute walking up, 7 per minute walking down. Doesn't sound like much, does it? But if you were to spend just ten minutes a day walking up and down the stairs of your apartment building, office, or shopping center, you could be burning an extra 85 calories a day with minimal effort. Some people add stairs to their day during a lunch break, or do a quick walk up and down during television commercials. I try to fit stair climbing in between seeing patients or when walking from my office over to the hospital.

People who climb stairs more frequently seem to reap the most benefits. A provocative study by the World Health Organization found an inverse relationship between people's body mass index and the apartment building floor they live on. People living on the fourth floor weigh less, on average, than people living on the ground floor. Even a few extra flights of stairs per day can help you burn an extra 50 calories per week—that's a slice of bread, some butter on your toast, or a small skim latte. And once you become more comfortable doing it, climbing stairs can become a source of pride as you open the stairwell door, glancing casually over at the masses pressing repeatedly on the elevator button. That's when you take them two at a time.

Solution #93
Walk During Breaks at Work

Walking is the easiest, most natural, and most effective way to incorporate activity into your life without stopping at a gym, setting aside extra time, or putting too much stress on your joints and muscles. Not everyone will be able to walk for thirty minutes a day, but it is a good goal. The advantage to breaking down walking into segments is that it becomes more manageable, especially for people with orthopedic or cardiovascular limitations. New data also suggest that small spurts of activity throughout the day may be more effective than getting your exercise all at once. The goal is thirty minutes, five times a week.

Most people take a lunch break of some kind at work—for some it is just twenty minutes and for others it can last up to an hour. And, like all of us, you know the feeling of trying to return to a desk, the truck, or wherever you need to be after your stomach is full. Your body is telling you it is naptime and your boss is telling you there are still five more hours to go.

Increase your energy level and make your lunchtime or any break time active. In a sense, a lunch break is recess for adults, when you get to take a rest from work and do something for yourself. For many people, this has evolved from the literal coffee break or personal phone call to an Internet break or Facebook status update. Go for a walk instead with one or several of your colleagues. Or if you just want a little time away from office politics, grab your iPod and go on your own.

Walking at the workplace not only makes sense, but it actually has been proven to help people lose weight. Many walking programs on job sites have resulted in better fitness and real weight loss for participants. For example, one study of a work-based walking program found that 93 percent of the participants lost weight. Talk to your employer about starting a wellness committee to integrate walking into break time, to create a community of walkers, and add some accountability to keep you motivated.

Most people should burn about 100 calories after walking for half an hour. Walk with a purpose. Listening to music or walking with coworkers can make the time pass more quickly, and will result in your walking faster and for greater distances. Taking a real break from your computer makes you feel refreshed and more energetic for the rest of the day. How's *that* for a status update?

FLEX Solutions

FLEX Solution #94
Walk After Dinner

After a long day at work or taking care of your kids at home, dinner is ideally a time to relax and catch up while enjoying a meal. But for many people today, dinner can be more stressful than the day leading up to it. You rush to grab takeout or throw together some random leftovers from the night before, and family time takes a back seat to texting at the table or cleaning your tomato sauce off the ceiling. But regardless of when you eat or how you eat your evening meal, the time afterward is a great time to spend together as a family or as a couple. And if you live alone, the time after you eat is a great opportunity to choose between the screen and the street.

Go for a walk after dinner. Commit yourself to once a week—weekends are sometimes easier. Just twenty minutes of strolling at a comfortable pace together will be enough to get caught up on your kids' latest exploits or your spouse's trials and tribulations at home or at work. Or if you go by yourself, it offers a chance for introspection and alone time. In just twenty minutes you can burn from 50 to 100 calories, which adds up if you keep it going. Take the time to reconnect with your family or yourself. You probably need it.

FLEX Solution #95

Walk Your Dog Every Day

In exchange for providing companionship, emotional support, and occasionally your slippers, dogs require a lot of attention and exercise to be happy. Many parents have their children walk the dog—part of the "responsibility" of having a pet, and also known as "so I don't have to." But each time your kids walk the dog—maybe just fifteen minutes twice a day—you are missing out on an opportunity to get outside, clear your head, and burn some calories without realizing it.

This was actually studied in a fitness campaign called Active Family, Active Dog. Seven diverse families with very different lifestyles were each paired with a dog and were asked to care for it for a period of six weeks. All the participants reported lower blood pressure readings at the end of the study, and all the families reported being happier after caring for their dogs. One reason for being happy was that they all lost weight. The seven families lost a combined fifty-five pounds in the short six-week period—this averaged about two to four pounds per adult involved. Given that you can burn at least 100 calories in the twenty minutes it takes to get Spot to do his business, it seems that the time is well spent.

FLEX Solution #96

Walk Before You Shop

Many Americans make a weekly or biweekly trip to Target, Costco, or the local shopping mall—one-stop shopping, lower prices, and plenty of parking bring advantages to suburban shoppers and people who live in more rural areas. One of the obvious features of big-box stores is . . . the big box. The combination of ample square footage and frequent visits sets the stage for a walking Solution that you knew was coming. Walk the store. The entire store. Not as part of your browsing or as you look for the best deal on chicken or diapers, but as an act unto itself. Burn calories before spending a single dime. You can easily log a quarter mile with one lap around the store. But avoid doing the Wal-Mart Walk— that absentminded zombie stroll with vacant stare that we are all prone to as we browse the aisles aimlessly. Walk with a purpose. You are trying to lose weight, after all.

If you have difficulty walking long distances, grab a cart and use it for support—no one will know the difference. You can even do your walk after you have picked all your items so that you get even more benefit from pushing the heavier cart along. If you like to go shopping with others, that works too. Pick a distance or pick a time and stick with it for a month. Then double it the following month. And double it again the third month. By the end of three months, you will be getting more exercise than you were before. But just hold on to your credit card.

LIVE

Solution #97

Make Grocery Shopping a Healthier Exercise

Grocery shopping is your opportunity to be in control of what you and your family eat. Consider these five steps to use shopping to help you lose weight.

1. **Do the shopping yourself.** If your spouse is buying bonbons and frozen French fries, that is what you are going to be stuck eating. You need to have a sit-down and go over your goals together, or you need to start making the trip by yourself.

2. **Eat before you shop,** and avoid having snacks and coffee drinks while shopping. And that goes for the candy in the check-out line too.

3. **Consider shopping online.** Many larger grocery stores will deliver for free or will waive the delivery charge if you spend a certain amount of money, buy a specific brand of diapers, or just prove yourself to be a loyal customer. One study found that after just eight weeks of food delivery, overweight individuals had fewer food items overall in their homes, and fewer high-fat foods, than those who shopped in the store. More home deliveries were correlated with more weight loss. It seems that the time that you spend ordering online gives you an opportunity to make better choices with fewer spur-of-the-moment decisions.

4. **Shop locally.** Living near a grocery store is associated with a lower risk of being overweight. In fact, for every grocery store within one kilometer of your home, there is an 11 percent reduction in the overall risk. You are more likely to walk than drive if you buy groceries close to your home. Also,

you are less likely to buy bulk groceries. When you buy only what you are going to eat for a couple of days, you lean toward buying fresh vegetables and just the staples rather than two-liter bottles of sugary soda and family-sized boxes of cookies.

5. **Stick to the list.** Plan your meals ahead of time. Healthier breakfast cereals. Whole wheat breads. More fish. More vegetables. Less juice. Less soda. And once you have determined which groceries you need, stick to that list when you enter the store. If you don't purchase items that are not on the list, you will not be able to eat them. And research suggests that a healthier food pantry leads to a healthier you.

Solution #98

Outsmart the Supermarket

People who design grocery stores think that they are smarter than us. It is no coincidence that dairy is in the back, candy is in the front, and finding the bakery section requires a compass. Supermarket layouts have been designed to make it difficult to find the things that you need by forcing you to meander through never-ending aisles of things that you may ultimately decide that you *want*. You end up spending money on impulse purchases when all you needed was a quart of milk.

But you can outsmart the supermarket to make healthy choices as well. When you walk into the store, head directly to the produce—it is typically on the side of the store near the entrance. It is close to the door because produce is profitable, so use this to your advantage and stock up here first. Do not be distracted by other items—salad dressings and baked goods sometimes sneak their way into this area. Then swing around the back of the store, where you will find dairy items. Make the frozen foods aisle (typically in the center of the store) your last stop on the way to the cash register, because this is where many processed, high-carbohydrate items are kept. And remember, candy and gum can tempt you at the checkout line, but they are not typically kept at the self-service checkout. You will save time by shopping more efficiently, and you won't be tempted to buy on the spur of the moment.

Solution #99
Buy Canned Fruits and Vegetables Without Additional Ingredients

Additives and preservatives are everywhere. But even if you are not going organic, it is worthwhile to think about what else might be in your can of food. Sugar and salt are commonly used as preservatives or for added flavor in canned foods, and corn syrup can sneak its way into the container as well. Do not let added calories ruin your fruits and vegetables. Eating canned foods can be less expensive as well as more practical, especially during colder weather when fresh options are harder to find. Just don't choose canned food that is higher in calories than it needs to be. Examine the nutrition label and look for canned fruits and vegetables with no added ingredients.

Solution #100
Read Food Labels

Nutrition labels are there for a reason: it's the law. But the reason for the law is that they give you the facts about the calories, fat, carbohydrates, and salt in the food you are purchasing. And that information can help you make better decisions. The first step is reading the label. Many people

Nutrition Facts		
Serving Size 2 tbsp (32g)		
Servings Per Container 16		
Amount Per Serving		
Calories 10	Calories from Fat 0	
		% Daily Value*
Total Fat 0g		0%
Saturated Fat 0g		0%
Trans Fat 0g		
Cholesterol 0mg		0%
Sodium 95mg		4%
Total Carbohydrate 2g		1%
Dietary Fiber 1g		4%
Sugars 1g		
Protein 0g		
Vitamin A 6%	•	Vitamin C 10%
Calcium 0%	•	Iron 0%

*Percent Daily Values are based on a 2,000 calorie diet. Your daily values may be higher or lower depending on your calorie needs:

are understandably intimidated by nutrition labels. But if you break them down, they are pretty straightforward. Let's focus on the information that will help you eat healthy and lose weight. Start by looking at the serving size, calories, fat, cholesterol, and sodium.

1. **Serving Size.** This is possibly the most important bit of information you will find, and it is listed first! The key thing here is recognizing what a serving size means: four cookies, nine chips, half the bottle—you get the idea. Then look at the number of servings in the bottle, can, or box and try to figure out how much you are going to eat or drink at one sitting. Because the information about fat, calories, and cholesterol won't mean a thing if you are consuming the entire contents. You do not have to commit to the recommended serving size, but you should use that information to understand the impact of eating *your* typical serving.

2. **Calories.** Remember that this refers to the number of calories *per serving*. You need to multiply this by the number of servings you plan to eat or drink at one time.

3. **The bad stuff.** Minimize fat, cholesterol, and sodium. Avoid trans fats entirely and look for low amounts of saturated fats in anything you eat and drink. Use the Percentage Daily Values to guide you—lower is better. Understand the meaning of terms like "low fat" and "cholesterol free" on labels, and remember that if a food is "free" of one thing, it may be "full" of another.

WHAT YOU READ	WHAT YOU GET (PER SERVING)
Calorie free	Less than 5 calories
Low calorie	Less than 40 calories
Light	One-third fewer calories
Low fat	3 g or less
Reduced fat	25% reduction
Reduced sugar	25% reduction
Reduced cholesterol	25% reduction
Cholesterol free	Less than 2 mg cholesterol and less than 3 g saturated fat

As helpful as they can be, food labels are useless if you do not read them. One research study found that most people use only the advertising catchwords on the front of the box ("Low Fat!" "Healthy!") to make purchasing decisions, rather than read the nutrition label. But if they turn the box and read the fine print, they start to make better decisions. People who know the most about nutrition are *twenty-five times* more likely to meet recommendations for fruit, vegetable, and fat intake than those who know the least.

Individuals with medically restricted diets have been watching their sodium and fat intake for years, but what about you? Reading nutritional information at the time of purchase influences 80 percent of people to change their food choices. And the result? Reading food labels is associated with eating less fat per day, as well as eating more servings of fruits and vegetables. The impact of choosing low-fat foods is huge in the long run, resulting in fewer calories that you need to burn. Every second you spend looking at food labels as you walk down the aisle makes your time on the treadmill that much more efficient.

Solution #101

Don't Eat from the Restaurant Breadbasket

Restaurants want to make customers happy. And one way they placate us is by distracting us from the inevitable wait while they cook our food. Hello, breadbasket. And while having a slice of high-fiber, low-sodium bread would be a good way to start your meal, the scones and muffins you get in restaurants are not baked with your diet in mind.

Restaurant bread is generally high in calories and low in fiber—it will not fill you up as much as other foods. Also, we tend to eat bread to pass the time at restaurants before the food arrives, and tend *not* to really "count" it as part of our dinner, and this can lead to eating too much. When you consider that a typical breadbasket might include four to eight servings, the numbers add up quickly.

Breadbasket Item	Calories
Melba toast	60
Oyster crackers	60
Whole wheat dinner roll	100
Italian bread	100
Sourdough bread	100
Breadstick	100
French bread roll	125
Pita bread	150
Bran muffin	300
Blueberry muffin	350

Consider some strategies for reducing the breadbasket's impact on your diet. Ask for the breadbasket to be half filled, or take just one item and then have the waiter remove the basket. Turn down the butter and request healthier olive oil. But all of this requires willpower. It may just be easier to ask your waiter not to bring the basket to the table at all. Just say no . . . to appetizer muffins, buttery croissants, and hearty slices of "home-baked" bread. Say no to mini-loaves, mini-cakes, and mini-buns.

The typical restaurant customer eats at least two breadbasket items per meal. Do that and it will run you at least 300 calories each time you go out. It is estimated that 40 percent of people eat out at least three times per week. Think about those business lunches with clients or meals at family restaurants on the weekend—that's a lot of bread. Try multiplying the number of breadbaskets you come in contact with each month by 300 calories, and enjoy the savings in turning them away.

Solution #102

Ask Questions in Restaurants

People are sometimes intimidated by ordering in restaurants. After the server tries to sell you the daily special, you are on the spot. It is not uncommon to make a last-minute decision while a family member is ordering. And then there is the ultimate display of uncertainty: "What's *your* favorite thing on the menu?" But when you are trying to lose weight, you shouldn't care what the server likes to eat—there are better questions that you could be asking. Ask the following three questions when you eat out and you are guaranteed to cut calories and improve nutrition.

1. **How is the food prepared?** The menu can be deceiving. Terms like "crispy," "battered," and "poached in oil" are all more appetizing ways of saying that something is fried. Get it out on the table and make sure you understand how your food is being prepared. Ask what kind of oil is being used (olive oil is a lot healthier than goose fat). This gives you an opportunity to ask for alternatives, like baking or broiling, that will significantly reduce the fat and calories.

2. **What are the ingredients?** Sometimes the menu does not contain the amount of detail that you need. Ingredients like butter, eggs, and bacon, and additives like MSG can enhance food texture and taste, but they can also add unwanted calories and fat or otherwise contribute to weight gain. They can

be introduced into foods like stews, casseroles, and beans without being obvious. Ask about them and see if the chef can make the dish without them.

3. **May I make a special request?** Nobody likes to give the server a hard time. But it is your money, and ultimately your health. This is the time to ask for steamed vegetables instead of fries, salad dressing on the side, and no mayonnaise.

....
: **FLEX** Solutions :
....

FLEX Solution #103

When You Buy in Bulk, Store in Servings

For people who live in the suburbs or shop for a larger family, it is much more practical to grocery shop less frequently and buy more. Big-box stores like Costco and Sam's Club reward buying in bulk with lower prices, so it is no surprise that so many shoppers load up the car and bring home huge quantities of paper towels, detergent, and hamburger buns. But larger containers of food—like chips and pretzels—do have a hidden cost. Despite a lower price at time of purchase, they cause "portion distortion" at snack time. Buy an industrial-sized box of reclosable sandwich bags during the same shopping trip, and take a few minutes to separate your snacks into individual servings. This way you will not miscalculate when you are hungry, and you will create a small obstacle to consuming too much at one sitting.

FLEX Solution #104

Avoid All-You-Can-Eat Restaurants

There are only a few reasons why you should find yourself looking at your reflection in the sneeze glass at an all-you-eat buffet—you have kids, you are in Vegas, or you are planning to break every rule in the book.

Buffets exist to tempt us into grabbing an éclair even though we are still building a salad or piling up a vertically challenged mélange of hash browns and Chinese stir-fry—and that's just on the first trip. As noted previously, research shows that the more variety we have in our diet, the more difficult it can be to lose weight. The buffet is a case in point.

It is extremely difficult to make good choices at an all-you-can-eat restaurant or buffet. While typically there is a salad and soup option, the buffet is designed to have you try as many things as possible, and it is priced accordingly. In order to get your money's worth, you can easily consume a day's worth of calories over the course of one meal.

Avoiding all-you-can-eat options is one way to eliminate the temptation to gorge yourself. But if circumstance (kids *or* Vegas) cannot be avoided, there are a few tricks you can use to curb the damage. Walk the length of the buffet table before selecting anything—it will remind you to eat the foods you should be eating instead of picking randomly at everything under a heat lamp. Choose a smaller plate; there are typically appetizer-sized plates and larger dinner plates that you can choose from at the beginning of the line. Limit yourself to the smaller plates and therefore smaller servings. Finally, limit your trips. You do not need to make separate trips for Italian food, Chinese food, the carving station, and the side dishes. If it can't all fit on one plate, then it shouldn't be stuffed into your stomach. One plate for salad, one for your entrée, and one for dessert is all you need. Another trick is to choose things you rarely get a chance to eat. There is no point in filling up on burgers or pizza when you can try a vegetable couscous or seared salmon that you can't get just anywhere. Dine adventurously, but remember that "all-you-can-eat" is a description, not a mandate.

FLEX Solution #105

Give Drive-throughs the Drive-by

Since In-N-Out Burger built its first drive-through restaurant in 1948 in Baldwin Park, California, the concept has spread throughout America and the world like a grease fire, with thousands of drive-through restaurants scattered along highways as well as in cities and small towns. As you know, drive-throughs are basically confined to fast-food restaurants. So if you place a moratorium on drive-throughs, you will make fast food a whole lot less convenient and will take away the spontaneity that leaves you "supersized." The simple Solution is to avoid them entirely.

FLEX Solution #106

Share an Entrée When You Go Out to Eat

Willpower has two parts; your plan and your behavior. Solutions turn words into action. There are the *Do This* and the *Don't Do That* Solutions, and then there are the *Jedi Mind Trick* Solutions that have you do one thing in order to change other behaviors without realizing it (for example, using small plates or starting a food diary).

This Solution, on the other hand, provides a simple way of decreasing your caloric intake by 50 percent without changing what you are eating. *Share.* Because if you do not have your own hamburger, you will not eat an entire hamburger. Same goes for burritos, steak, fish, and shepherd's pie. It doesn't matter what you're ordering—just share it with your dining partner.

So simple. You will decrease your calories by half and cut the cost of eating out significantly in the process—even if they do charge you two bucks to split the order. So get your two bucks' worth by asking the server to split the order onto two plates in the kitchen—the deed is done even before the food arrives on the table. You can also employ the "I split, you choose" method at the table to avoid any arguing over who got more green beans.

Sharing with your dining partners gets them in on the act too. We know that people lose more weight when they lose it together. And there is nothing more romantic than sharing. With the money you will save, maybe you can start eating out more often.

FLEX Solution #107

Avoid MSG

Monosodium glutamate, or MSG, is a flavor enhancer used widely in processed foods. A recent study found that individuals who consume higher levels of MSG are three times more likely to be overweight than people who do not consume MSG at all. This effect appears to be independent of exercise or even total calories consumed.

The reason behind this relationship is not well understood. While it could be argued that MSG improves food flavor and therefore increases the amount we eat, some argue that MSG impacts the way we metabolize fat. MSG typically is used in highly processed foods, which are also associated with weight gain.

Given that MSG does not have nutritional value, avoiding it is a good general health practice that may also help you lose weight, if only because it will lead you to avoid some processed foods. Look carefully at the ingredients of common foods like barbecue sauce, salad dressing, bouillon cubes, and snack foods. Seasoning mixtures, which many people use in order to avoid using table salt, are also a common source of MSG. And don't forget about soy sauce.

Food Products and Additives Containing MSG

Calcium caseinate
Corn oil
Hydrolyzed protein
Hydrolyzed yeast
Sodium caseinate
Textured protein
Yeast extract

FLEX Solution #108

Make Mexican Food Healthier

When Americans go out for Mexican food, visions of burritos the size of a baby's arm and oversized terra-cotta plates buried under a melted mass of cheese, beans, and orange rice fill our collective consciousness as well as our stomachs. But it does not have to be that way.

The basic components of Mexican cooking actually have some pretty healthy attributes. Beans are high in protein and fiber. Tomatoes, corn, and chilies are rich in nutrients. Spices rev you up. Interestingly, heart disease is less common among Hispanic Americans than among non-Hispanic Caucasians. But the paradox is that obesity is increasingly more common in Hispanic circles. Many explanations circulate, but one possibility is that the Americanization of Mexican food has impacted the people who eat it the most.

As Mexican cuisine has evolved to meet American expectations, so have the portion sizes. Meals served at many family restaurants regularly contain over 1,500 calories—a day's worth for some people. That makes going to one a great time to share. Skip the tortilla chips. People can easily consume 500 calories in chips at one sitting. When ordering a predinner drink, consider a regular margarita or a light beer rather than a flavored margarita—they tend to be lower in carbohydrates. If you are making drinks at home, take a look at Bethenny Frankel's Skinnygirl margarita recipe (www.bethenny.com/skinny_margarita .htm) with about half the calories. Corn tortillas have half the calories of flour tortillas. Quesadillas are filled with cheese, fajitas with grilled meat. Choose chicken over *carnitas*. Remember, *refried beans have been fried more than once*—choose black beans instead. And that last-minute decision to add cheese, guacamole, or sour cream can add 500 calories to a single meal.

FLEX Solution #109

Ask for a Doggy Bag When You Order Your Meal

Restaurant serving sizes have gotten out of control. You frequently read about gargantuan portions of appetizers, entrées—even salads—that provide you with over half (if not all!) of your recommended daily amounts of fat, salt, or calories. Studies do show that portion sizes have increased in fast-food and family restaurants. It does not cost a restaurant much money to give you extra food. The restaurant ends up making a profit, and you somehow feel as though you are getting a deal. And the enormous portion that arrives at your place setting seems to justify the wait.

Some diet books have highlighted the nutritional quagmire that occurs when you are given 1,400 calories at one sitting. Usually the first recommendation is to go somewhere else and avoid these restaurants (and temptations) entirely. But the reality—especially for people who travel for work or have young children—is that dining options can be pretty limited. The second recommendation is to order something else. This can work if you are familiar with the menu or if "healthy choices" are listed, with nutritional information. But sometimes you want to order what you like. What's a diner to do?

Pack it up. Take it home. Save the rest for lunch tomorrow. Most restaurants will be happy to do this for you. But the key is timing. When you have already eaten all but one of your mini-egg-roll appetizers, it is too late. Same goes for that last chicken finger or scrap of chicken pot pie. And oftentimes the remainder on your plate is not particularly appetizing or has soaked up so much sauce that you probably don't even want it.

So get your doggy bag first. At the time you order, ask your server to bring you half your entrée or appetizer and pack the rest separately—ask to have it brought to you when you receive your check. This works especially well for appetizers or even pasta. You have just reduced your portion size—and calorie intake—by half (sometimes more than 500 calories in a meal), and you did not have to exercise restraint. Too easy. And you will have lunch for tomorrow too.

FLEX Solution #110

Order a Better Pizza

Pizza's actually healthy for you if you don't eat too much of it.

—JOHN SCHNATTER, FOUNDER OF PAPA JOHN'S

Everybody loves pizza, but even Papa John recognizes that there can be too much of a good thing. Make pizza good for you in seven easy steps.

1. **Order thin-crust pizza.** Avoid deep-dish or pan pizza (unless you are in Chicago, of course) and reduce your calorie intake considerably. For example, one large slice of Pizza Hut's Thin 'N Crispy pizza has about 90 fewer calories than the deep-dish option. That is over 700 calories per pizza.

2. **Ask to have your pizza cut into twice the usual number of slices.** If you would typically eat four slices of pizza, the idea of consuming eight slices may slow you down and result in your eating less pizza. If you are able to eat just one-half slice less, you will cut 150 calories.

3. **Blot your pizza.** Use a paper napkin to blot the visible oil off the surface of your pizza. One gram of fat is 9 calories and takes up about a quarter of a teaspoon—you can absorb up to 40 calories per slice.

4. **Limit yourself to one meat topping.** Many restaurant menus offer "combination" options with multiple meats on one pizza. One large slice of Pizza Hut's Meat Lover's pizza offers about one-half of the total recommended daily amount of sodium. You can decrease the amount of salt and calories by about 25 percent (about 110 calories per slice, and nearly 1,000 calories per pizza) if you enjoy a slice with only pepperoni instead. Realistically, you cannot detect the subtleties

of each taste if you have three or four different kinds of meat on a pizza anyway.

5. **Bulk up on vegetables.** Vegetables are good for you, and they fill you up. So put them on your pizza. And pizzas with vegetable toppings are often prepared with less cheese. For example, a large slice of Pizza Hut's Veggie Lover's pizza has 30 fewer calories than a cheese slice.

6. **No appetizer pizza.** No dessert pizza. No salad pizza. Just eat the pizza that's for dinner.

7. **Put away your leftovers first.** Decide before you eat how much you are going to eat. Put away the extra slices for tomorrow, so that you will not be tempted to have an extra slice now.

FLEX Solution #111

Think Outside the Bun

Sorry, this Solution has nothing to do with Taco Bell. But people often do minimize the caloric impact of eating the buns, breads, and pitas that keep their sandwiches together. Bread does not contribute significantly to the taste of the filling, so you can do without it. I personally have a tough time eating a sandwich or burger totally naked, but I have noticed that, much of the time, the bread or bun is oversized as compared to the filling. You can reduce your carbohydrate intake significantly by trimming the extra bread around the edges of the sandwich. It doesn't look as pretty, but it still tastes better than an iceberg lettuce wrap. Another alternative is to ask for the sandwich or burger open-faced. You will cut the carbohydrates in half without feeling as though you are really depriving yourself.

FLEX Solution #112

Go Grocery Shopping Without Your Kids

Children are wonderful. But anyone who has ever taken a child to a supermarket knows that it can be a risky endeavor. Not only are kids distracting when you are trying to read nutrition labels or compare items, but they tend to get pretty bored. Boredom turns into tantrums, and tantrums turn into Pop-Tarts. Children have the unique ability to make their parents buy candy, sugary cereal, or an extra cookie at the bakery counter in order to make the rest of the shopping trip go more smoothly. Call it love or call it extortion, it works either way. Don't think you will outsmart them with a piece of fruit or some baby-cut carrots—they do this for a *living*. And the problem is that their gain is your loss. When you ask the person in the bakery section if there are any broken cookies to sample, it seems pretty harmless to have a taste yourself. And every opened box of crackers or cereal leaves the rest of the box for you to snack on. If you can, leave the kids at home so that you can make good choices for you *and* your family. But if you think you can control yourself (and your kids!), you can Flex this Solution by bringing the kids along and creating an educational opportunity for them. You can be a good role model by teaching them about the healthy foods that fill your basket.

4.

YOUR WAY

You have your way. I have my way. As for the right
way, the correct way, and the only way, it does not
exist.

—Friedrich Nietzsche

Y ou have had a busy five weeks. You started by spending
two weeks getting hydrated, supplemented, stretched, and
mindful. You then spent twenty-one days rebooting your system and made some significant, incremental changes in the
way you eat, drink, exercise, act, and live.

Now comes the interesting part. Solutions come in different flavors.
There were the changes that you could make Today, and the ones you
should follow Every Day, but now it is time to do things *Your* Way.
Welcome to nearly one hundred more lifestyle hacks, changes, and Solutions that you can use to take things to the next level. They are all Flex
Solutions. Look for more outside-the-box thinking and some original
approaches sprinkled among additional ways of retooling your nutrition
and activity. Your goal is to choose just ten.

The Solutions are organized into the five categories you have already
seen in the Every Day Solutions—Eat, Drink, Exercise, Act, and Live.
Pick two Solutions from each section and follow them. Do not be
discouraged if some do not interest you or will not fit into your lifestyle. The point is that not all of them will. *Your* Way is different from

someone else's. Choose only those Solutions that you want to try. And if you find later on that you want to explore others, you can switch them out—but make sure that you are following at least ten in total. In three weeks, you will develop ten new habits that you will take with you. I suspect that, in the end, you will choose even more. *Your* Way.

THE *YOUR* WAY SOLUTIONS

Eat

113. Fast.
114. Eat slowly.
115. Substitute lower-calorie and lower-fat cheese for what you are already buying.
116. Eat at least 25 grams of fiber each day.
117. Eat more protein at breakfast.
118. Add some spice.
119. Substitute fruit for cooking oil.
120. Ask for your sandwiches without cheese.
121. Use cooking spray.
122. Substitute for sour cream.
123. Stop using margarine and butter in cooking or as spreads.
124. Order smaller serving sizes.
125. *Hari hachi bu* one meal a day.
126. Clean out your freezer.
127. Know your serving size and eat one less.
128. Avoid white starches.
129. Order the children's meal at fast-food restaurants.
130. Consume fewer than 2,400 milligrams of sodium a day.
131. Eat your grapefruit.
132. Avoid anything with high-fructose corn syrup.
133. Eat rhubarb.
134. Don't use cheese as a garnish.
135. Skim oil and starch off the top when cooking.
136. Eat your largest meal of the day from a smaller plate.

137. Use bowls for snacks.
138. Pack your spouse's lunch.
139. Shop at a farmers' market once a week.
140. Splurge once a week on anything you like.

Drink

141. Don't use nondairy creamer.
142. Add ice.
143. Order wine by the glass.
144. Drink light beer.
145. Drink coffee instead of cocoa.
146. Drink additional water before going out to eat.
147. Cut out sugar substitutes.

Exercise

148. Move your exercise to the early morning.
149. Bicycle.
150. Join a sports league.
151. Run every other day.
152. Exercise during commercials.
153. Swim.
154. Add interval training to your workout.
155. Take up yoga.
156. Increase your time exercising by just one minute each week, and exercise faster.
157. Practice tai chi.
158. Race.
159. Dance.
160. Run barefoot.

Act

161. Get up, Get NEAT.
162. Take care of your own lawn.
163. Use trekking or walking poles.
164. Use hand weights while you walk.

Live

165. Meditate.
166. Use a financial incentive to reward your weight loss.
167. Play active video games.
168. Stop smoking marijuana.
169. Try acupuncture.
170. Change your commute.
171. Get hypnotized.
172. Chew gum four times a day.
173. Just watch the movie.
174. Change your environment to avoid temptation.
175. Reduce the amount of time you spend watching television.
176. Laugh for thirty minutes a day.
177. Wait twenty minutes before eating snacks or eating dessert.
178. Use blue.
179. Brighten your environment.
180. Listen to music while you exercise.
181. Brush your teeth after meals.
182. Turn off the Food Channel.
183. Buy a headset.
184. Say no to samples.
185. Bring your own airplane snacks.
186. Set the alarm on your computer.
187. Give your seat to someone else.
188. Kiss your partner ten times a day.
189. Don't order room service.
190. There's an app for that.
191. Clean out your closet.
192. Start a garden.
193. Make social outings active rather than food oriented.
194. Lobby to get menu calorie labeling in your area.
195. Use chopsticks.
196. Photograph your food.
197. Those shoes are made for walking.

198. See yourself thin.
199. Fill in the blank.
200. Count your blessings.

EAT

Solution #113

Fast

Fasting might seem like the ultimate diet plan or debacle, depending on who you ask. The obvious problem is that it cannot be sustained for very long. But anyone who celebrates Yom Kippur or Ramadan will tell you that it can be done in a controlled setting without much of an issue. It is estimated that as many as 14 percent of Americans have tried fasting to lose weight.

There is already evidence in animal research that periods of fasting are associated with a slower aging process. And Mormons who fast once a month have been observed to have a lower risk of heart disease. But before you even consider fasting, you should clear it with your doctor. Diabetics and women who are pregnant or breast-feeding should generally not participate in a diet that incorporates fasting.

For the appropriate person, fasting for short periods of time appears to be both safe and effective when done the right way. Fasting for more than a day, however, may not yield any additional benefit, and it will result in your feeling low in energy. The key to a safe one-day fast is to maintain hydration and avoid caffeine and alcohol. Plan your fast for a day on which you do not plan to do strenuous exercise. Avoid fasting to punish yourself for diet mistakes; conversely, try not to reward yourself with food the following day for a job well done. Consider doing a one-day fast once every three weeks. Start at eight o'clock on the first night, fast the following day and night while maintaining hydration, and eat a healthy breakfast at eight o'clock the next morning.

One argument against fasting is the possibility that the person will be starving on the day after and will try to make up for lost time by overeating, and therefore will cancel out any benefit from the fast. But research shows that after the person eats a large breakfast this effect goes away and does not impact meal choices throughout the day. A one-day fast is associated with weight loss of 1 to 2 percent of total body weight. Intermittent fasting over a period of months is also associated with sustained weight loss. Some studies have also suggested that brief periods of fasting can be associated with an enhanced sense of well-being and mild euphoria. Also, evidence points toward beneficial long-term effects on the brain and heart. Not a bad side effect.

Solution #114

Eat Slowly

Chew with your mouth closed. Clean your plate. And slow down. Even though your mother was just trying to help improve your manners, there may be some actual benefit to eating slowly as far as weight loss is concerned.

The idea is that if you eat slowly, your stomach will signal to your brain that you are full, and you will take in fewer calories overall. While we already know that consistently eating until you are full doubles your likelihood of being overweight, research also suggests that eating *slowly* may reduce your risk by half. If you make a point of eating slowly, you can reduce your caloric intake by 70 to 100 in a given meal while feeling fuller than if you ate more quickly.

This strategy of eating slowly to maintain a healthy body weight is well regarded in Japanese culture. And some people believe that slower eating partially explains the "French paradox," the phenomenon that French people are generally thinner than Americans despite their significant intake of cheese and other foods high in saturated fat.

The Slow Food Movement

1. Chew each bite five times.
2. Put down your utensil between bites.
3. Serve your food in courses.
4. Have a sip of water between bites.

5. Turn off the television.
6. Talk about politics at the dinner table.

So, how can you eat slowly? Well, a fork with an electronic timer was patented almost fifteen years ago and does not seem to have gained much traction in the market at this point, so you may be on your own. You can start with chewing—chew at least four or five times with each bite, instead of "inhaling" your food. Consider putting the fork down between bites. Talk with your family at the dinner table. Present your food as multiple courses rather than all on one plate (and serve the vegetable before the meat). Try chopsticks. Drink water. Turn off the television. Put on some soft, soothing music. Try dinner, for starters. And chew with your mouth closed. And that advice about always cleaning your plate? We'll have to talk about *that* one, Mom.

Solution #115
Substitute Lower-Calorie and Lower-Fat Cheese for What You Are Already Buying

Many people enjoy cheese, and one of the toughest things about dieting is the thought of giving it up. But cheese can be part of a weight-loss program if good choices are made in the dairy aisle. People assume that all cheeses are equally high in calories and saturated fats, but that is not actually the case. Here are some guidelines to use when shopping for cheese at the grocery store.

1. **Buy cheeses made from skim or low-fat milk.** While Cheddar cheese is 30 to 40 percent fat, cheese made from skim milk or low-fat milk can have a fat content of less than 15 percent. Hard cheese generally has more fat than soft cheese, but lower-fat or even fat-free options are still available.

2. **Consider naturally lower-fat cheeses**—like ricotta, cottage cheese, and Gouda.

3. **Choose cheeses that are generally low in salt**—like Swiss or Parmigiano-Reggiano—for even greater weight-loss benefits.

4. **Consider buying low-lactose cheeses**—like feta or aged Gruyère. Some dieters have more gas because they are eating more vegetables than usual or are lactose-intolerant. Choosing cheeses like these might help.

Do a quick comparison between these options and your usual cheese the next time you are shopping. You will be surprised at how easily you can cut calories and fat without sacrificing much else.

Solution #116
Eat at Least 25 Grams of Fiber Each Day

A research study recently found that two factors account for 90 percent of the variation in people's body weight worldwide. Job-related physical activity is one, and dietary fiber is the other. So if you are not ready to change jobs quite yet, maybe it is time to start thinking about getting more fiber in your diet.

Fiber comes in two types: soluble and insoluble. The soluble kind dissolves in water—think oat bran, fruits and vegetables, nuts and beans. Water-soluble fiber helps to prevent your body from reabsorbing bile acids, and this can help lower your cholesterol without medication. Insoluble fiber (wheat bran, whole wheat bread, most vegetables) does not dissolve in water, so it absorbs water in your stomach and intestines and keeps you "regular." Not a bad thing either. This is why a diet high in fiber may be lower in calories but will still fill you up.

The American Heart Association recommends that adults eat 25 to 30 grams of fiber (both soluble and insoluble) daily. The typical American gets about half that amount. Whereas low fiber intake is associated with obesity, increased intake of dietary fiber from fruits and vegetables is associated with weight loss. If you can increase your total daily fiber intake to bring it in line with the recommendations of the American Heart Association, you can expect to lose at least a pound a month.

But let's be clear. I am not recommending that you chug Metamucil or take other over-the-counter bulk fibers. Although these agents can be beneficial in some settings, the concern is that taking fiber as a supplement can result in significant dehydration without offering nutritional value. Instead consider bulking up your daily fiber intake with fruits and vegetables and other sources of dietary fiber. Here are a few high-fiber foods to get you started.

Food	Fiber (g)
1 cup brown rice	2.5
1 banana	3.0
1 cup strawberries	3.3
1 cup cauliflower	3.4
1 apple	3.7
1 pear	4.0
1 cup canned minestrone soup	5.0
1 cup broccoli	6.0
1 cup raisin bran	7.0
½ cup Fiber One cereal	11.9

You may already be consuming enough fiber, so it is worthwhile to examine your diet and determine whether you should be adding more. After you have kept a food diary for a week, use a Web resource like GlobalRPh (www.globalrph.com/fiber_content.htm) to calculate your average daily fiber intake. By making small adjustments to portion sizes or by adding certain fruits, vegetables, and grains, you can easily determine how you can increase your intake to recommended levels. Incorporating the American Heart Association's daily fiber recommendations into your diet is a commitment, but doing so will benefit you in many ways beyond weight loss, from improvement in cholesterol levels to potential reduction in your risk for certain types of cancer. Not to mention making you regular.

Solution #117

Eat More Protein at Breakfast

Protein fills you up more than carbohydrates and makes you less likely to crave calories midmorning or eat a larger lunch. Eggs are a great Solution, but few people can eat them every day. Think about more creative ways to introduce some protein into your breakfast. Tofu, black beans, lean turkey, and nuts can all be incorporated into the most important meal of the day. Protein-fortified breakfast cereals like Kashi GoLean are a great option for the traditionalist. And don't forget about Greek yogurt, peanut butter, and soy nut butter.

Solution #118

Add Some Spice

There are lots of great reasons to add spices to your food. While there is no single "magic spice bullet" that will guarantee significant weight loss, making a sustained effort to incorporate multiple seasonings into your food may help you lose weight. Spices have some features that make them useful as weight-loss adjuncts.

1. **They make food taste more interesting.** Many people find it challenging to make the switch from salty, fried foods to healthier food because of a perception that healthier food just won't taste as good. By adding oregano, pepper, and garlic, for example, you can fool your taste buds into thinking they are experiencing a higher-calorie treat.

2. **They can reduce your appetite.** Cooking with garlic and spicy chilies is a great way to make your first serving more satisfying and keep you from reaching for seconds.

3. **They can increase your metabolic rate**—by as much as 10 percent, for short periods of time. Capsaicin (found in chilies) and capsiate (found in paprika and red peppers) may have this effect.

4. **They can help reduce fat absorption.** Ginger, fenugreek, and garlic all have this property.

Using these ingredients in your cooking will help you enjoy your food more while eating less of it. In restaurants, asking your server to make your food spicy is easy enough, and the chef usually appreciates the opportunity to prepare a more authentic-tasting dish.

Solution #119
Substitute Fruit for Cooking Oil

We can learn a lot from how we feed our babies. Once they graduate to solid food, we give them a steady diet of pureed fruits and vegetables, with very limited amounts of meat and oil. While baby food on its own certainly is not appetizing to an adult, we can actually use things like mashed banana, pureed prunes, applesauce, and canned pumpkin in our own diet to increase our fiber intake, lower our total calories, and lose weight.

Try substituting an equal amount of mashed or pureed apples or pears for cooking oil when you bake at home. You will reduce the amount of fat significantly—think 1,000 calories in a batch of brownies. Keep in mind that food with less oil will cook more quickly, so check the oven at least five minutes before the end of the recommended cooking time to make sure that you do not overcook. A new market for baby food?

Solution #120

Ask for Your Sandwiches without Cheese

Although we often expect cheese when we order a hamburger, eat at Subway, or make our own turkey sandwiches, the truth is that cheese adds less in taste than it does in calories. One slice of cheddar has about 6 grams of saturated fat and more than 100 calories. To put this in perspective, someone taking in 2,000 calories a day should be limiting himself or herself to fewer than 16 grams of saturated fat daily.

You easily can drop 100 calories from your lunch just by having your sandwich without cheese. In a month, you can drop a pound's worth of calories this way without changing anything else about what you are eating. If you think that this will detract significantly from the taste, try this experiment. Go to Subway and ask for your favorite sandwich, but say that you want cheese placed only on half of it. Start eating from either end, and you will quickly realize that the cheese did not make much of a difference.

Solution #121

Use Cooking Spray

Most people use some oil when they cook. It is something that you do not usually think about as you add it to the frying pan. But oil is not about adding taste to your food, it is more about keeping it from sticking to the pan. And sometimes fruit puree just won't do the job—you need some oil to make certain dishes work. That's where cooking spray comes in. Cooking spray is a great alternative to bottled oils, but there are some things you have to keep in mind so that you get the most benefit.

1. **Cooking spray is still oil.** So it's not as though you have discovered an alternative ingredient for cooking that will save

you fat and calories. This stuff is the same stuff you are trying to avoid. The key difference is in delivery and quantity.

2. **Advertisements can be misleading.** Remember that food companies have a nice deal going with the Food and Drug Administration. If you put less than half a gram of fat into a serving of a particular product, you are legally allowed to say that the product is fat free. So the next time you see a "Fat Free!" label on a canister of olive oil cooking spray, think again.

3. **You always use more than one serving.** Because cooking spray is aerosolized, manufacturers can define a serving size as a spray of just *one-third of a second*. But spraying so briefly is basically impossible to do in the real world. Many people coat the bottom of a pan as if they were applying varnish to a chair. Just remember, three seconds of spraying is almost ten servings.

Despite these shortcomings, cooking spray is still a great alternative to slathering butter or margarine in your pan, or adding globs of oil. A one-second spray delivers about a gram of fat—fewer than 10 calories. It takes about a second to say "Flex Diet" (or any other phrase that is slightly less embarrassing). Contrast this to a tablespoon of butter, margarine, or oil, which has *more than 10 grams* of fat and more than 100 calories. Also consider that many people cook with the same amount of butter or oil, regardless of how much food they are cooking or how many people they are serving. This can mean a lot of fat and calories. Your vegetables will not know the difference, but your pants will. I recommend using canola or olive oil cooking spray.

Solution #122

Substitute for Sour Cream

Sour cream is not just for baked potatoes and Mexican food. People use it frequently in baking, soups, and dips. But there are some easy substitutions that will significantly lower fat and calories. Try reduced-fat or nonfat sour cream for starters, and if you do not like the flavor, you can try nonfat or low-fat yogurt, cottage cheese, or even evaporated milk with just a splash of lemon juice.

Solution #123

Stop Using Margarine and Butter in Cooking or as Spreads

Whether it is on bagels, English muffins, toast, pancakes, waffles, baked potatoes, or even corn, people are still using butter. This may be the result of a backlash of public sentiment about spreads, instigated partly by doctors and scientists, and partly by people's desire to stick with a seemingly more natural alternative.

Butter has obviously been enjoyed for years. But doctors and government agencies started to crack down on our use of butter once researchers and nutritionists learned more about the dangers of saturated fats and the associated increased risk of heart disease. Conveniently, margarine was available as a pretty tasty alternative, and many people felt that they were doing something heart-healthy by making the switch. If you are still one of those people, prepare to be schooled on spreads.

It is true that margarine is lower in saturated fat. Unfortunately, it usually turns out to have trans fat, which is now recognized as even worse for us than saturated fat. This was not as well understood back when the butter-or-margarine debate was at its height, and many of us made the switch without much evidence except for the common sense that less saturated fat meant healthier food.

So margarine ends up not being a great option either. And you may already know that both margarine and butter have similar numbers of calories, so you are not going to get much of a weight-loss impact from making a switch. This makes things challenging, even for those of us who are not using stick margarine (the trans-fatty one) anymore, but are using the newer trans-fat-free alternatives. Lower-calorie or trans-fat-free margarines are definitely an option. But people often use more than the serving size of one tablespoon, and that makes it hard to cut calories significantly.

If you can train your taste buds to enjoy an ear of corn or your morning waffles without either of them, that is the best way to go. But if you can't help yourself, then at least consider the newer vegetable oil spreads and olive oil spreads, as well as the plant stanol spreads that have been clinically proven to lower your cholesterol while livening up your baked potato. While you will not eliminate many calories with the switch, you will at least be eating healthy fats that are better for your heart. You can even make olive oil spread at home by freezing a container of olive oil until it hardens, and then putting it into the refrigerator until it reaches spreadable consistency. Also consider low-sugar and low-calorie fruit spreads, or honey, which has about half the calories of butter or margarine.

If You Can't Believe It's Not a Great Idea to Eat Butter, then maybe it is time to reconsider all those waffles, pancakes, baked potatoes, and bagels too.

Solution #124
Order Smaller Serving Sizes

For restaurants, food is cheap. So when you order a larger serving of food and pay a higher price, it seems like a fair deal—but to the restaurant it is an even *better* deal. And you pay in more ways than one.

For example, when you are at the movies, you frequently pay for the larger size of popcorn or soft drink, because it seems like you are getting more for your money. Prices are set at places like Starbucks or McDonald's in such a way as to convince you to buy the larger item—so that you feel like you're getting a deal. And research also shows that when we order larger sizes in an effort to stretch our money further, we end up eating and drinking more than we really want or need.

Ordering the smaller serving size will save you money in the long term and calories in the short term. Let's consider the difference in calories between a small and a medium size (or lunch and entrée size) in some food and beverage items you might encounter outside your home. Even if you only eat out once every few weeks, it will add up quickly.

Calorie Difference: Smaller vs. Larger Size

Food/Beverage (smaller size)	Difference (calories)
Starbucks 2% latte	40
Cola beverage	60
Wendy's Chocolate Frosty	90
McDonald's French fries	150
Applebee's Santa Fe Chicken Salad	300
Movie popcorn	380
Burger King Hamburger (vs. Whopper)	390

Ordering smaller will let you continue to enjoy the foods and drinks you already are enjoying, and you will still have enough to keep you satisfied. Take the money you will save and buy some smaller-sized outfits instead.

Solution #125

Hari Hachi Bu One Meal a Day

Japanese people pretty much live forever. It's true! Japan has more centenarians than any other country in the world—and for obvious reasons everyone wants to know why. While it is true that Japanese cuisine highlights fish and downplays dairy, two lesser-known cultural concepts may account for much of Japanese longevity and general good health.

The first is the idea of *nuchi gusui,* an Okinawan term that means "life's medicine," or "food as medicine." This is the concept that food is something not only to be enjoyed, but also to be thought about critically as actual medicine that is being taken into the body. When you pay attention to the health impact of food as you eat it—its sugar and saturated fats, not to mention its beneficial vitamins and nutrients—it makes it harder to stare down a basket of deep-fried potato skins without being at least a little embarrassed. Thinking of food as medicine makes you more mindful of every choice you make. As you become more thoughtful and recognize everything you eat and drink as a *true* choice, you may ultimately make better choices.

One such choice could be adopting the Japanese practice of *hari hachi bu. Hari hachi bu* is the practice of eating until you are 80 percent full. It's that simple. Whereas "food as medicine" teaches us to think carefully about each food choice and how it will impact our body and our health, *hari hachi bu* is more about quantity. Studies do suggest that we can eat less than the quantity that makes us "full" and still be satisfied. Japanese people traditionally practice restraint as a matter of course, and they use this discipline to their body's advantage with respect to calories. We know from animal studies that consuming fewer calories is associated with a longer and healthier life. This would appear to apply to human beings as well, when you consider the number of hundred-year-old Japanese folks hanging around.

How do you practice *hari hachi bu*? Try one meal at a time. Most of us can forecast about how much we will eat at a given meal, whether it is three slices of pizza, one or two helpings of mashed potatoes, or the full bag of chips. Choose one meal each day and make a determined effort to eat only until you are 80 percent full. Leave 20 percent on the plate or in the bag or the box. And then put it away until another time. You will be surprised at how much easier it is to limit calories when you are thinking about just one meal rather than a full day, a week, or a month at a time. All the same, the calories will add up.

Solution #126

Clean Out Your Freezer

Once a month, your freezer needs a good cleaning. But this type of cleaning focuses on its contents. Frozen fruits and vegetables offer convenient ways to stock up on vitamins and fiber at any time of day, whatever the season. But frozen premade foods and snacks are typically highly processed and have too much salt, sugar, and fat. While microwave meals can be an exception, look closely at the ingredients. Choose only those meals that apply the "2-4-8" rule—20 grams of protein, fewer than 400 calories, and fewer than 800 milligrams of sodium per serving. Clean everything else out of the freezer and you will be amazed at how easy it is to avoid frozen snacks, appetizers, and desserts.

Solution #127

Know Your Serving Size and Eat One Less

This Solution has a similar goal—portion control—to *hari hachi bu* but approaches it differently. We know ourselves pretty well. For example, I know that I would eat four slices of pizza for dinner, but only two at lunch. I also know that I tend to order a "medium" of whatever beverage is offered. I will eat one and a half egg rolls as an appetizer at a Chinese restaurant if my wife lets me. Two strips of bacon if it is for breakfast— one for the initial taste and the second because I know I shouldn't.

After a lifetime of feeding yourself, you get into a rhythm, fueled less by hunger and more by expectation and habit. You eat that last slice of pizza or scoop up another plate at the breakfast buffet not because you are still hungry—the first half of your meal took care of that. You do it because, well, *that's what you do.*

This Solution is less about healthy food choices and more about quantity. An interesting study published in *The New England Journal of Medicine* compared four diet strategies, from low-fat to low-carbohydrate to everything in between, and found that weight loss did not differ significantly among the different approaches. Weight-loss success correlated simply with caloric intake. Whereas many studies have debated the relative merits of different strategies, this report highlights the importance of portion control. It all comes down to calories.

We know already that large shifts in the way you live your dietary life are difficult to sustain—and are not very much fun. As long as you can make small dents in the number of calories you consume each day, you will lose weight over time. As they say in dietary politics, it's the calories, stupid. Instead of always obsessing about *what* you eat, concentrate on eating *less*.

So start with one. One less cup. One smaller size. One less cookie. Approach *each meal* with a plan for the item or quantity you will have one less of, and soon you will have at least one less pound to show for it. As you keep your food diary, make a point of indicating which items you could have one less of. You will be amazed at how many calories you will cut with a bit more mindfulness.

For example, at breakfast, if you always have three slices of toast, just eat two. If you typically have two slices of cheese on your turkey sandwich at lunch, just eat one. And if you grab two biscuits from the breadbasket, eat two burgers off the grill, or have a few cookies before you go to bed at night . . . You get the idea. Enjoy *what* you enjoy already, but enjoy one less.

Solution #128
Avoid White Starches

A simple way to make good food decisions is just to look before you eat. If you are about to eat a starch, consider its color. White starches in pasta, white bread, white rice, and potatoes are refined and have a higher glycemic index rating than brown starches. High-glycemic-index foods will cause you to have higher peaks in blood sugar and can wreak havoc on your insulin regulation. This is why diabetics are generally instructed to avoid these foods. Brown starches like those in whole grain breads and brown rice are associated with weight loss, in contrast to their lighter-looking counterparts. Interestingly, white starches are particularly associated with belly fat—a feature of metabolic syndrome and correlated with heart disease. Buy brown starches for home cooking, and make a point of avoiding white starches in restaurants. Many restaurants have recognized the benefit of brown starches, and will prepare brown rice at your request. Remember to look for "whole wheat flour" or "whole-grain flour" as the first ingredient—"wheat flour" and "enriched unbleached flour" could sneak white flour into the recipe without your knowing it.

Solution #129

Order the Children's Meal at Fast-food Restaurants

The best Solution is to avoid fast-food restaurants entirely. But for many people who spend a lot of time on the road, fast-food restaurants are just a reality. And we all know that their convenience comes at a steep price in calories.

There are always healthier alternatives in a given fast-food chain's menu, but the question is whether you will have all this information at your fingertips the next time you are standing in line or entering the drive-through. There are multiple iPhone applications that can help you out, but if you do not have the time, patience, or iPhone to make this happen, there is always the children's meal.

Whereas regular restaurants typically require the presence of a child before allowing an adult to order a children's meal, fast-food restaurants typically are not as picky. Ordering the kids' option makes a possibly more complicated food-ordering decision pretty straightforward, and it will automatically save you calories as compared to a similar adult-sized option.

For example, a Happy Meal at McDonald's will run about 480 calories (just the burger and fries), whereas ordering a Quarter Pounder and medium fries off the adult menu will run about 790 calories. While you can obviously just order smaller portions off the regular menu, the children's option is already a well-defined, complete meal.

And you get a toy too.

Solution #130

Consume Fewer Than 2,400 Milligrams of Sodium a Day

Cardiologists are constantly asking their patients to reduce their sodium intake. We know that taking in more sodium is associated with higher blood pressure. Adopting a lower-sodium diet will not only bring down blood pressure, but will also reduce symptoms of heart disease like shortness of breath or swelling. This is because sodium attracts water and carries it wherever it goes. If you consume lots of sodium, the volume of water in your bloodstream and tissues goes up, and this can put stress on your heart and your blood vessels.

Following a lower-sodium diet therefore results in less fluid retention, which does impact your water weight. But the reason for having less sodium in your diet is not to reduce your water weight. Obviously, water is not fat—and sodium has no calories. So where is the benefit in the long term?

Let's think about where you get your sodium. Only about 11 percent of the sodium in a typical American diet comes from salt added to food during cooking, salt added at the table, or condiments like soy sauce or ketchup. But 77 percent comes from eating prepared or processed foods like canned vegetables, luncheon meats, frozen foods, and prepared soups. Even if a food does not taste terribly salty (bagels can have over 400 milligrams of sodium), the presence of ingredients like monosodium glutamate (MSG), baking soda and baking powder, and nitrites should tip you off—you will be surprised at the sodium content of many foods if you read the nutrition labels.

And it turns out that most processed foods tend to be lower in fiber and higher in calories than foods with naturally lower amounts of sodium—which also happen to be better foods for weight loss. Lowering your sodium intake to recommended limits will change how you shop for food. You will move away from less healthy foods and toward fresh vegetables, frozen items with no added sugar, and higher-quality prepared foods. It is not a coincidence that many of my patients who adopt a lower-sodium diet lose weight without that purpose in mind.

Solution #131

Eat Your Grapefruit

Most fad diets are based upon some science. For every Cigarette Diet, Tapeworm Diet, and Drinking Man's Diet out there, you will find a weight-loss program highlighting the potential benefits of acai berries, peppermint, or even grapefruit. Although grapefruit is known to interact with a number of medications, it also is a great weight-loss food to incorporate into a balanced diet.

Grapefruit is somewhat unique among citrus fruits in that it reduces insulin levels, which means that you will be less likely to crave other sweet treats. Grapefruit is also a fruit with high water content, so it will fill you up, especially if you eat it before a meal.

One study of grapefruit and weight loss found that eating grapefruit or even taking grapefruit capsules was associated with losing at least three pounds. If you are not crazy about eating grapefruit every day, then capsules are a safe, somewhat more expensive choice. Remember to discuss this Solution first with your doctor to make sure that the grapefruit will not significantly interact with any medicines you might be taking.

Solution #132

Avoid Anything with High-fructose Corn Syrup

High-fructose corn syrup is a sweetener that is used in place of sugar in everything from soft drinks to salad dressing, and even bread and soup. When many people think of sugar substitutes, thoughts turn to coffee sweeteners and diet soda, but high-fructose corn syrup is in a majority of processed foods.

Many scientists attribute the surge in obesity to increasing consumption of high-fructose corn syrup; some also argue that it increases the risk of diabetes and abnormal cholesterol levels. There are also recent concerns that high-fructose corn syrup made in the United States may contain mercury. The small incremental increase in calories provided by fructose adds up when you consider all the foods that contain it. Because of its lower price, high-fructose corn syrup may also be partially responsible for the oversizing of bottled soda and packaged baked goods. And we may crave it even more than sugar.

Eliminating high-fructose corn syrup from your diet is easier said than done. But if you start avoiding packaged or processed foods in which it is a significant ingredient, you may find that you are spending more time in the fruits and vegetables section of the supermarket. And that would be really sweet.

Solution #133
Eat Rhubarb

Weight loss in a pie. Sounds pretty good, right? Although we associate rhubarb with pies and jam, it is actually a vegetable. And like many vegetables, rhubarb is low in carbohydrates and high in fiber, and so it is a great weight-loss food. In addition, it is rich in the compound anthraquinone, which may reduce fat absorption in the intestines and help rhubarb function as a mild laxative. You can use rhubarb as a tasty substitute for fruits like strawberries in pies and jams, or you can add it raw to yogurt or fruit salad to keep you feeling fuller for longer.

Solution #134
Don't Use Cheese as a Garnish

Many people use cheese as an afterthought—they sprinkle it on chili, eggs, and pasta for some added texture and flavor. Just a few tablespoons of parmesan or a quarter cup of mozzarella has about 100 calories that you can easily do without. Estimates of cheese consumption in the United States suggest that we have at least tripled our intake since the 1950s—more cheese correlates with the increasing prevalence of obesity. Cheese is incorporated into processed foods and baked goods more than ever. Although it can be difficult to reduce your consumption of cheese when it crops up in processed foods, you can choose to reduce your daily calories and saturated fat intake by not using cheese a garnish.

Solution #135

Skim Oil and Starch off the Top When Cooking

We all know that oil and water do not mix. So take advantage of this chemistry tidbit and apply it to your soups, stews, and stir-fries. During the cooking process or even after the food has been served, you can frequently find a few tablespoons of oil that have not soaked into your vegetables or meat. Use a ladle or your soup spoon to skim it off and set it aside. A tablespoon of oil is about 100 calories, so this can make a significant difference over time.

You can do the same thing with starch. You may notice that when you boil pasta or rice there is a white film that rises to the surface. This is starch, which is another way of saying sugar. You can get rid of it easily with a spoon or ladle, and it will help you avoid some calories without changing the taste. Skimming off the top is an effortless trick that is guaranteed to reduce your overall calorie intake.

Solution #136

Eat Your Largest Meal of the Day from a Smaller Plate

Portion control is obviously not a new concept. But many people do not realize that serving sizes of common food items have been increasing steadily for decades. The largest portions are found in fast-food restaurants, more than at other restaurants or at home. And the magnitude of the increases is what is most unsettling. A traditional fast-food meal of a hamburger, fries, and a soda will run you at least 200 calories more than it did when you were a kid. If only your metabolism increased at that rate too.

It would be one thing if we could leave that last French fry on the plate, or put down the sandwich when our hunger has been satisfied. But it is not that simple. The power of convenience is apparently superior to willpower. Shocking, right? More food on the plate ultimately translates into more food in our stomachs. One study found that when restaurants increase portion sizes by half, restaurant customers will eat about 50 percent more than they will when smaller portions are served. Some have even speculated that the lower rates of obesity in France as compared to America may be the result of American portion sizes gone wild. We should let them eat *our* cake too.

But research also shows that you can decrease your portion sizes by 25 percent and feel just as full as you did with the larger serving—your mind and stomach can't tell the difference. This has led some to suggest that using a ten-inch dinner plate (rather than the twelve- or fourteen-inch size we typically use) will cause you to serve yourself about 20 percent less food than you normally would. One study actually found that the average person lost two pounds in a month just by using a smaller plate for dinner. Ten-inch plates should be available anywhere that housewares are sold. Consider stocking up on smaller serving bowls, smaller serving spoons, and smaller cereal bowls too.

Solution #137
Use Bowls for Snacks

As we can see from the effect of plate size on calories consumed at meals, visual cues have an obvious impact on the amount we eat. So let's use this information to learn about how using bowls for snacks can make a difference.

Your appetite doesn't really know what it is doing sometimes. Despite the reality that the best, most satisfying, most *delicious* bite is always the first one, after that bite some reptilian urge then takes over and you mechanically finish whatever is in front of you. While it is sometimes hard to exercise willpower, it isn't so hard to limit what is in front of you in the first place.

If you have any doubts about whether people eat until the container is empty, consider the results of a research study done on soup consumption. Subjects ate from a bowl of soup that was rigged to *refill itself* from beneath the table in an imperceptible way. Participants ended up eating on average, *73 percent more* soup than those who ate from a normal bowl, but did not believe that they were any fuller or had eaten any more than the people eating from a normal bowl.

Take the bottomless-soup-bowl concept and apply it to a box of cookies or graham crackers or a bag of chips. The container does not provide you with any visual cue to how much you have eaten—so you end up eating a lot more than you might realize.

Use a dedicated snack bowl for all snacks. Preferably a small one. Pick a bowl that will hold a single serving of whatever snack you ordinarily enjoy. If you pick a bowl large enough to allow you to share with others, you will not know how much you are eating. Choosing a smaller bowl for yourself is just as important. This was illustrated in a study of ice cream bowls and serving spoons. A group of nutrition experts were fooled by larger bowls into eating 31 percent more ice cream than other participants using smaller ones. And if nutrition experts can be influenced so easily, then we do not have a chance.

Being a successful dieter or healthy eater is apparently not just about what you know. It is about what your body expects. Changing your body's expectations is one of the most challenging mental aspects of eating right. But you can change those expectations without even realizing it by putting them in a new context with visual cues. And research also shows that if you change your behaviors first, you will tend to change your attitudes to fit them. So for starters, fit them into a bowl.

Solution #138

Pack Your Spouse's Lunch

You may find it easier to make good choices if you make fewer of them. The morning ritual of packing lunches for everyone typically falls on one person. But if you can get your partner, spouse, or roommate to help you out, it's a nice idea to consider packing each other's lunch. It eliminates the temptation to add an extra slice of cheese to your sandwich or put a cookie at the bottom of the bag, and it keeps you accountable to someone else. The best part? You get to write a note.

Solution #139

Shop at a Farmers' Market Once a Week

Farmers' markets are everywhere. As people have become more interested in what they eat, farmers' markets have provided a link between city appetites and farm products. Farmers increase their customer base through direct sales, and consumers get access to local foods and fresh produce. Shopping at a farmers' market once a week will prompt you to stock up on wonderful varieties of fruits and vegetables that might look a little more appetizing than the produce you find sweating under bright lights and sprinklers at your big-box supermarket. And shopping weekly will help you plan meals—the foods are not frozen and do not have preservatives, so you will need to eat them soon.

Many people will be surprised to find how many farmers' markets are available in their area. The United States Department of Agriculture estimates that there are about 4,800 farmers' markets in the United States. Check out their website at http://apps.ams.usda.gov/farmersmarkets to see what is available in your city or town. There are fourteen in my own hometown of Portland, Oregon. You will be surprised to find what is near you.

Solution #140

Splurge Once a Week on Anything You Like

As you have learned, success in dieting is no miracle. Success comes with focus, education, and constant attention to lifestyle. After a week of hard work, many people feel that they have earned a little freedom to treat themselves on the weekend. And research shows that allowing yourself this latitude actually helps you stay on track the rest of the time.

That is why many of the Solutions in this book are designed around a five-day workweek, with the understanding that most people have different eating habits and schedules on the weekend. This is not to say that you should go back to all your old behaviors, but you can start by choosing one thing each weekend that you really know you will enjoy. This might be a particular dish at dinner, a dessert you love, or even just lazing around the house.

By choosing and planning for a particular indulgence, you accomplish a few things. First, you will not feel guilty. Guilt about messing up their diet is one of the major reasons why people quit on the weekend and start again on some future Monday that keeps being pushed back. But if you plan for those nachos or that slice of cheesecake, it becomes part of your plan. You are in control. There is no setback. And it will be easier for you to continue your diet at the following meal.

Second, you will maintain control of your intake. Choosing one 500-calorie dessert or burger with all the fixings is a very different decision than mindlessly adding 100 calories here or there with mayonnaise, soft drinks, and whole-milk lattes. Do not go back on the small changes that got you this far.

Finally, planning a splurge makes you less likely to give up your diet for the sake of a birthday, anniversary, or other special event, and keeps you focused during your regular days. And in the same way that the thought of Saturday can get a lot of people through a week in the office, your expectation of a treat on the weekend can keep you with the program throughout the week.

The weekend allows you to refocus and review your Solutions again on paper and in your mind. It is the time to buy those healthy groceries, clean out your pantry, prepare some homemade soup that will last you through the week, and maybe even get in a long bicycle ride. The weekend reminds you to pace yourself, and the thought of Monday means that you are in this for the long run. Enjoying a treat is part of that.

Sure, it's not like you are creating the world in six days each week. You are only trying to lose a couple of pounds by manipulating your subconscious, changing your outlook, and modifying your diet and activity. Sometimes I'm not sure which is harder.

DRINK

Solution #141

Don't Use Nondairy Creamer

Go to any office lunchroom across the country and you will find it. Nondairy creamer. Sounds innocent enough. For the lactose intolerant, it would seem like a nice option. And for coffee drinkers who do not have a refrigerator available, the powdered nondairy creamers can be pretty convenient. But our use of nondairy creamer at home or at work is a prime example of how serving sizes mean different things to different people—and nondairy creamer means too many calories for too many people.

How do you decide how much nondairy creamer you are going to add to your coffee? Do you pull out a tablespoon (the recommended serving size) and measure it out, or do you just pour it into your cup and stop when it turns your coffee the right color? Consider that each tablespoon of nondairy creamer runs 10 to 20 calories compared to 5 calories in a tablespoon of nonfat milk. Adding a liberal amount of nondairy creamer to your cup of coffee could mean 50 calories per cup.

One concern with nondairy creamer in particular is people's perception of its health benefits—or rather lack of risks as compared to milk products. The nutrition label may show zero grams of fat, but remember that if *one serving* of a food item has less than one-half gram of fat, the food can be labeled as having no fat (the same goes for trans fats). For example, Nestlé Coffee-Mate Fat Free Original Powder and Fat Free Original Liquid each list "partially hydrogenated" oil as the second or third ingredient (after corn syrup solids). This means trans fats, and while the label does state in small print "Adds a trivial amount of fat," if you end up using two or three servings at once and multiply that by four or five cups of coffee a day . . . you are consuming significant trans fats in addition to calories.

If you can commit to making a change in your brew, you can shave a surprising number of calories with relatively little effort. Use less sugar. Avoid sugar substitutes. Avoid nondairy creamer, but if you have to use it, use one serving at a time. And if you really want to make a difference? Drink it black.

Solution #142
Add Ice

As long as you are drinking water every day, you may as well make it work for you more efficiently. Or better yet, you should work for *it*. When you drink ice-cold water, you burn a small number of calories to warm it to your body temperature.

Let's think about the definition of a calorie. First, remember that the calories we commonly talk about in terms of diet and exercise are actually misnamed. The more accurate name for these is *kilo*calories—each kilocalorie is a thousand *actual* calories. For whatever reason, the "kilo" prefix has been dropped from common usage. We will use the right measurements for the purpose of understanding how adding ice to your drink can be beneficial.

A real calorie is the amount of energy it takes to increase the temperature of one kilogram of water by 1 degree Celsius. An eight-ounce glass of water weighs about 235 grams, or 0.235 kilograms. An ice-cold glass of water is at zero degrees Celsius, and your body temperature runs about 37 degrees Celsius. So if you multiply 0.235 grams by 37 degrees, you are burning about 8.7 real calories when you drink an ice-cold glass of water.

It may not seem like much of a Solution. But when you consider drinking six glasses of ice-cold water a day, you could potentially burn more than 50 real calories a day without any additional effort. While this isn't a substitute for good food choices or getting some exercise, 50 calories is 50 calories. So cool it.

Solution #143
Order Wine by the Glass

When you are eating out at a nice restaurant and feel the urge to enjoy some wine, limit your serving by ordering just a glass. Buying a bottle costs less per glass, but in order to get your money's worth, you need to drink the whole thing. Even if you split the bottle with a dining partner, this means that you will drink two or three glasses before you are done. At about 100 calories per glass, you can save yourself some 200 calories while dining out if you stop at one.

You can use the same strategy when enjoying wine at home by pouring yourself a glass and then corking the bottle and storing it away. If you leave the unopened bottle on the table, you might find yourself refilling your glass as a matter of habit rather than because you really want to drink more. The calories will add up either way.

Solution #144
Drink Light Beer

Talk about sacrifice . . . time to dig deep and switch to light beer. This is understandably a difficult Solution for many people. Despite the encouraging advertisements, it's hard to get excited about Diet Beer. But in all fairness to the beer companies, there are more choices than ever before, and some are actually pretty decent. While the big domestic brews tend to dominate this market, there are also some nice options from smaller, local breweries and foreign producers. They all offer a significant reduction in calories, and the newest brands are taking it even further. Combine with pong for a Light Beer Workout.

Light Beer vs. Regular Beer

Beer Solution	Light (calories/serving)	Regular (calories/serving)
Amstel Light	93	n/a
Budweiser Select 55	55	145
Budweiser Select	99	145
Coors Light	102	148
Corona Light	109	149
Sam Adams Light	119	160
Heineken Light	99	166
MGD 64	64	143
Michelob Ultra	95	155
Michelob Ultra Amber	114	155
Miller Lite	96	155
Sapporo Light	96	140
Yuengling Light	98	135

Solution #145

Drink Coffee Instead of Cocoa

Many people are concerned about the potential negative health effects of coffee, with respect to things like palpitations, nervousness, and heart arrhythmias. But it is reassuring to learn that a wealth of research on the subject has surprisingly come out in favor of coffee. In fact, some studies have even found that consistently drinking coffee may reduce the risk of both diabetes and Parkinson's disease. And while I might discourage people from drinking ten cups a day, modest intake does not appear to be associated with significant cardiac problems; in fact, there may actually be some benefit.

In addition to boosting your alertness, improving your mood, and providing a somehow legitimate excuse to take a break, coffee may have some attributes that benefit you as a dieter. First, as a liquid, it takes up space in your stomach that might otherwise be filled with a jelly doughnut. Some people do not like to drink water, but they can finish a pot of coffee without much of a problem.

Next, coffee boosts your metabolism and increases body-heat production (thermogenesis) so that you burn calories just a wee bit more efficiently. One study suggests a 7 percent increase in metabolic rate for three hours after a person drinks one cup of coffee, and another found that drinking coffee can burn an extra 150 calories over a twelve-hour period. While that might require six cups of coffee, drinking more reasonable amounts would be expected to produce a smaller but still significant effect.

Caffeine also serves as an appetite suppressant, as does the taste of coffee itself. The acidity can temporarily impact your taste buds and make other foods taste less appetizing. Ever wonder why you have coffee at the end of a meal rather than at the beginning at most restaurants?

Consider strategizing your coffee intake—space it at regular intervals instead of taking it as a huge dose in the early morning, and drink it before meals rather than afterward. Grabbing a cup of coffee (even decaf!) during breaks can also help remind you not to be eating something higher in calories. Iced coffee works just as well, if not slightly better, for reasons described in Solution #142.

Solution #146
Drink Additional Water Before Going Out to Eat

You should already be drinking six glasses of water a day. But when you are planning to go out for lunch or dinner, it is a good idea to drink one or two glasses of water before you leave the house or the office. Interestingly, the fluids we consume during meals do not tend to affect our appetite or ultimate calorie intake significantly. During the time it takes for our stomachs to signal to our brains that we are full, we have consumed more calories and done the damage. This is why eating a bowl of soup *before* a meal helps to reduce calories overall—the soup fills you up, and by the time the entrée arrives you have less of an appetite. Water works the same way. If you drink it before you set out, you will start to feel fuller by the time you sit down to the table. You may even order less food as a result of feeling less hungry. Drinking water at the table is also beneficial, but your best bet is to have water appease your hunger before you even place your order.

Solution #147
Cut Out Sugar Substitutes

You hopefully have already stopped drinking diet soda, but now it is time to tackle sugar substitutes in other drinks and foods you enjoy. The whole idea behind sugar substitutes is to help reduce calorie intake—this is why foods containing them often are labeled "diet." But for something to really be effective as a diet food, it has to help you reduce overall calorie intake, lose weight, and get healthier. Seems obvious, but sugar substitutes generally do not make the grade. While people with significant dental issues or diabetes mellitus may certainly benefit from sugar substitutes for obvious reasons, most other people do not.

The scientific evidence suggests that people who consume significant quantities of sugar substitutes may actually take in more calories overall than those who stick with just plain sugar. And people who go without either benefit the most. This is because sugar substitutes taste so much like sugar that they trick our minds and bodies—but only at first. Insulin levels increase in anticipation of a big sugar load, but when it does not arrive, blood sugar levels fall. This disruption in our sugar equilibrium makes us crave more sugar (i.e., glucose, metabolized from food) to set things right. Also, the seemingly good choice you made by drinking diet soda or adding a sugar substitute rather than sugar to your coffee may steer you toward an extra doughnut hole later as a reward. You may not be aware of it, but it happens.

In addition to being in diet soda, sugar substitutes commonly crop up in coffee drinks, and with the recent marketing push for stevia, expect to see them elsewhere. Remember the millions of free NutraSweet gumballs mailed to Americans in the mid-1980s in what was possibly the first viral marketing campaign?

But research on sugar substitutes continues, and the latest information is pretty provocative. Oligofructose, long used in Asia, was recently studied and found to be associated with no significant weight gain as compared to a placebo—but the exciting finding is that it was also associated with drops in cholesterol and blood pressure. If this appears to be a long-term effect, do not be surprised to see oligofructose listed as the next superfood. Or, at the very least, supersweetener.

EXERCISE

Solution #148

Move Your Exercise to the Early Morning

While getting adequate sleep is an essential part of any healthy weight-loss plan, there may be advantages to getting your exercise early in the day. The first is that you get it over with. There is nothing better than finishing nighttime rituals with your kids, or getting home after a hard day at work, and then settling down to relax with the knowledge that you have already taken care of possibly the toughest challenge of the day. The other possible advantage of morning exercise is more efficient fat burning. When you exercise on an empty stomach, your body does not have any stored sugars to provide fast energy to your working muscles, so you tend to burn proportionally more fat. When you exercise later in the day, you tend to burn more sugar. You will burn similar numbers of calories regardless of when you exercise, but you may experience different long-term results in your overall body composition if you exercise earlier in the day.

One concern about early-morning exercise is that you may be more prone to injury. Your body temperature is lower in the morning than in the afternoon, and this may increase the risk of injuring your muscles. Also, exercising later in the day gives you a chance to stretch out naturally over the course of the day, and some would argue that this decreases your risk of muscle injury. Regardless of how or when you exercise, it is always advisable to discuss it first with your doctor to make sure it is safe for you.

So set your alarm a half hour earlier and press the snooze button to feel that you have exercised your right to sleep. But then get up and burn some calories before starting the day.

Solution #149
Bicycle

Even though your old bicycle is gathering dust in the garage, cycling is still one of the best ways for you to get exercise, stay fit, *and* lose weight. Its advantages are obvious—cycling is low impact, making it a great choice for weekend warriors with bad knees. You can enjoy it together with your family or on your own. You can do it on vacation, or even while commuting to work. You can choose your route, your pace, and how long you are on the road. And for those days when the weather does not permit cycling outdoors, you can pick up an exercise bicycle for the cost of a few weeks' worth of groceries. Now all you have to do is use it.

Studies show that bicycle riders tend to be fit and trim. An interesting comparison of adults from North America, Europe, and Australia found that people who bicycled more (Europeans) had the lowest levels of obesity. Part of this geographic trend may be that Europeans tend to view walking and cycling as means of transportation rather than as exercise alone, and so both get incorporated more easily into a European lifestyle. More compact city centers and shorter work commutes facilitate this as well.

Active commuting may also be associated with a reduction in the risk of heart disease. It has been estimated that, to get this benefit, you need to be on your bicycle for just about ten minutes, twice a day. Even if you are not in a position to cycle to and from work—or if you do not have a regular commute—you can easily incorporate this amount of cycling into your day. It is even more convenient if you have an exercise bicycle at home. You will burn about 100 calories in fifteen minutes of cycling, whether you are stationary or not. Start at just fifteen minutes a day, but be consistent about it and get on the bike five times a week. Increase your workout by five minutes each week, so that you are cycling for thirty minutes, five times a week, at the end of your first month.

If you do not typically get much exercise, start out by just riding at a comfortable speed, stretching your legs and enjoying the scenery (or what's on television if you are inside). Having the exercise bicycle in your living room or bedroom will also motivate you to use it while you watch the news or your favorite reality show. After a few weeks, you can adjust the time and resistance to your legs' content.

Solution #150

Join a Sports League

Many adults trying to lose weight longingly remember their high school days as competitive swimmers, runners, and football players. The combination of youth's higher metabolism and lots of physical activity made calorie intake irrelevant. But after just a few years go by, we are amazed to find our athlete's body hidden under a few extra layers, even in summertime.

The good news is that those glory days do not have to be gone forever. Increasingly, adults are finding that joining a local sports league is a great way to commit to exercise on a regular schedule. And injecting some competition into your workout makes it a little more exciting than pressing the incline button on a treadmill. There are options for pretty much everyone, from flag football to volleyball to kickball to dodge ball, in addition to the standard softball league. You can find out about local offerings from people at work or at your nearest community center or place of worship. Online resources like www.sportsmonster.net and www.sportsvite.com as well as more local sites can also steer you in the right direction. Choose a season, pick a sport, and show up on time. Your teammates will be counting on you.

Solution #151

Run Every Other Day

Running does not cost anything, can be done nearly anywhere, and can be fun to pursue on your own or with a group. But losing weight by running has more to it than just lacing up your shoes. Emerging data suggest that higher-intensity, shorter-duration exercise may be even more effective for weight loss than slower, longer workouts. Try running for shorter distances, but increase your speed. Not only will your workout be more effective, but it will be more efficient too. As you train, keep an eye on your food diary simultaneously to make sure that you are not rewarding yourself for your hard work with a box of cookies after your workout. A runner's high, after all, can give you the munchies.

Solution #152

Exercise During Commercials

Digital video recorders are everywhere now, and they are used for two obvious purposes: to record television programs for later viewing, and to fast-forward through commercials. You end up watching more television than ever, but you do it more *efficiently*. But despite the technology, there will still be nights when you watch the news or your favorite reality shows in real time.

Let's focus on those two-minute segments of commercials that turn a forty-seven-minute program into an hour. A commercial break can be more than an invitation to buy a juicer or a ShamWOW—it can be an opportunity to get off your butt and do something. Get your heart rate up. Move around the house. Maybe even sweat.

Can you be active for two minutes and lose weight? Definitely. It turns out that you can burn 20 calories in two minutes pretty easily if you get intense about it. Don't have a treadmill or an exercise bicycle? No lap pool in your living room? See what you can burn during a commercial break:

Two minutes of sit-ups? .... 20 calories
Two minutes of push-ups? .... 20 calories
Two minutes of step-ups? .... 20 calories
Two minutes of fast stairs? .... 20 calories
Two minutes of jumping rope? .... 20 calories
Two minutes of shadow boxing? .... 20 calories
Two minutes of plyometrics? .... 20 calories
Two minutes of jogging in place? .... 20 calories

Get the idea? If you do something vigorous, even for just two minutes, you can burn about 20 calories depending on your body weight. (Heavier people actually burn *more* calories!) You know you're doing it right if you get your heart rate up and feel that slight bead of sweat on your brow as you settle down for the next tribal council. Twenty calories may not seem like a lot, when you consider that you need to burn at least 3,500 calories to lose a pound. But think about the average one-hour episode of *American Idol* (we're talking results show here). After waiting an hour to find out that the guy you knew was going to be voted off was in fact voted off (and sitting through yet another guest appearance by Clay Aiken), you have wasted about thirteen minutes (although some might argue it was more like an hour). So instead of wasting them, spend them. Just one hour of watching television could mean burning more than 100 calories. With that logic, if you watch the Oscars, you could fit into a smaller dress or pants size by the end of the show.

Just don't touch that remote. . . .

Solution #153

Swim

Many people are under the impression that if you swim for exercise, you will not lose any weight. This has possibly been sparked by the idea that we require body fat to insulate us in cold water, suggesting that swimming will help us pack on muscle without burning much fat.

But if you have ever watched the Summer Olympics, you will realize that either swimmers are practicing in boiling water, or swimming actually helps you keep in great shape. Michael Phelps has famously described taking in about 12,000 calories per day, so it would appear that swimming can keep off the pounds. Otherwise he would have gained about twenty-five of them by the time he won that eighth gold medal in 2008.

Swimming is a great option for people with arthritis or balance issues that can limit their ability to perform weight-bearing exercise. Water-based exercise can be done individually, but if you enjoy exercising with a group, multiple classes are available. For people who do not enjoy swimming but like being in a pool, just walking back and forth in the shallow end burns calories and aids weight loss.

Swimming can help you lose weight just as effectively as walking. Researchers have found that both walkers and swimmers can lose thirteen pounds in three months just from exercising three times a week.

Solution #154

Add Interval Training to Your Workout

It is easy to get into a pattern when you exercise. Once people motivate themselves to get to the gym, they usually have a pretty good idea of what they are going to do once they get there. It becomes a routine: set the treadmill to a comfortable speed or set the resistance on the exercise bike, put on the headphones, and zone out for the next half hour. But studies show that this is not the best approach if you are trying to lose weight by exercising.

Interval training is the concept of changing exercise intensity for predetermined periods of time within a workout. Exercise experts have found that the surge of adrenaline that occurs during the transition from lower-intensity to higher-intensity exercise may have an even greater benefit for burning fat and, ultimately, losing weight. In one study, participants either cycled for forty minutes at a steady pace or exercised for twenty minutes during which they alternated between eight-second sprints and twelve seconds at slow, gentle speeds. Despite exercising for only half the time, the interval trainers lost more weight and more body fat. The researchers speculated that adrenaline is released during these short sprints and targets fat cells.

Interval training is not limited to exercise bikes—you can do it on the treadmill, in the pool, on a rowing machine, or even walking around your neighborhood. Create a pattern for each minute in which you go slowly for forty seconds and then quickly for twenty seconds. Compare the way you feel after one of these workouts to your typical routine. You will burn more calories overall while saving time. And if you are able to do interval training throughout your typical workout, you have really won the game.

Solution #155

Take Up Yoga

Yoga uses stretching, stationary poses, and isometric exercises to burn calories in a uniquely low-impact way that makes it a great exercise option for nearly everyone. It is worth considering especially for people who are not comfortable exercising in public gyms or who have joint problems that limit their ability to exercise in other ways. It can be done nearly anywhere, inside or outside, and it does not require any expensive equipment. People can enjoy yoga by taking a class or by doing it at home using a DVD for guidance. Some well-reviewed DVDs include *Yoga Shakti; Power Yoga: Total Body Workout; Brian Kest's Power Yoga: Complete Collection;* and *Yoga Conditioning for Weight Loss.*

If you are considering yoga as a Solution, it is a good idea to get acquainted with the various types, so that you can get a better sense of how you could incorporate it into a weight-loss program. The many varieties of yoga make it a form of exercise that most people can enjoy, but keep in mind that the lower-intensity versions will not burn enough calories to make a significant weight-loss difference. Here are brief descriptions of the most common yoga styles with associated calories burned per hour and more conventional exercise forms (with higher impact on your joints) that might yield a similar result.

YOGA STYLE	WHAT YOU DO	CALORIES YOU BURN*	COMPARABLE ACTIVITY
Hatha	Stretching, breathing exercises, meditation	100–200	Light walking
Ashtanga	Faster paced, with emphasis on poses	200–300	Brisk walking
Vinyasa	Faster transitions between poses	400	Moderate bicycling
Bikram	Yoga performed in a room heated to 105°F	600	Jogging

Research shows that yoga is also associated with reduced stress, lower blood pressure, and improvement in control of diabetes. Part of this is related to weight loss, although some would argue that the deep breathing and meditative aspects provide additional value that makes yoga unique.

*Per hour

Solution #156

Increase Your Time Exercising by Just One Minute Each Week, and Exercise Faster

Interval training is just one way to make sure your exercise routine does not become *too* routine.

Many of my patients who exercise five or six times a week know their routines to the second, and can spout off information about time spent and heart rate achieved on the treadmill or the elliptical or stair-climbing machine. But plateaus occur naturally among people who exercise regularly. After a while, if you do the same thing every day, you begin to see fewer results from it. This is the reason why some exercise programs have you cross-train among different disciplines, including both aerobic and weight-bearing exercise.

Recognize your plateaus and turn them into slopes. Your challenge is simple. If you use exercise equipment, increase your pace and your duration of exercise by small increments. Just one-tenth of a mile per minute, and one extra minute each week. It does not sound like much, but small changes do add up.

For example, a 170-pound person who walks for twenty minutes at 3.0 mph will burn about 110 calories in the process of walking one mile. At the end of ten weeks, the same person will be walking for thirty minutes at 4.0 mph, which means two miles . . . and 200 calories. Changing the parameters of your exercise slowly will increase your endurance as well as exercise duration, which is associated with increased fat burning.

Solution #157

Practice Tai Chi

Can a billion Chinese be wrong?

Tai chi is a centuries-old discipline made up of beautifully choreographed sequences, described by some as "moving meditation." Its slow, fluid, graceful movements are performed in casual clothes, are low impact, and do not require special equipment. You may have seen people practicing this art in parks in the early morning. It looks pretty relaxing, but it is also surprisingly effective exercise.

Its benefits are achieved through a unique combination of mindfulness and slow, purposeful movements that isolate muscle groups and improve strength, balance, and coordination. Tai chi is an ideal exercise for young and old alike and has been shown to improve balance and strength as well as help older people live independently. For overweight individuals who are mostly sedentary, or people with knee or ankle pain, tai chi provides a low-impact option that is gentle on joints but still burns calories. Clinical studies have shown that it plays a role in fat reduction. But perhaps its greatest proven benefit is in lowering stress—which also helps in maintaining a healthy weight.

Tai chi classes are available at most health clubs, martial arts schools, and senior centers. And there are always the early mornings in the park. . . .

Solution #158

Race

Sign up. Pay the fee. Get a number.

If you have never committed to competing on a track, on the road, in the water, or on the trail, this is the time. Entering a race—of whatever type, and whatever distance—is a Solution that will jump-start so many parts of your life. The combination of competition and a specific goal will also lead you to incorporate Solutions where you did not even know you had them.

My first race was the result of a challenge made during my senior year of college. Two days later, I ran the Boston Marathon. I do not really recommend doing it that way. But that experience of meeting other runners along the way, hearing the high-pitched roar from the women's college campus along the route, and crossing the finish line inspired me to try different competitions, from sprint triathlons to mountain biking, and a few more marathons as well. I will always be an average competitor, but that is not the point. As with many things, completing the race is not the only goal—another is how you get there.

It can be hard for many of us to motivate ourselves to exercise. But when you create concrete goals for yourself rather than having open-enders, *and* you have committed the time and money to enter a race of whatever kind, you will be inspired to train. And the racing community is composed of people with so many levels of skill—the great news is that there will always be a person slower than you.

Check out websites like www.active.com and www.coolrunning.com to get started. You can find information about races in your area as well as training tips to keep you safe. Many people also enjoy joining a team-in-training with friends or work colleagues—a great way to raise money for an important cause and extend your commitment to others as you train. It also helps you get up at five in the morning to go for a run when you know that other people are counting on you to do the same.

Your degree of weight loss will depend on your starting point. Very overweight or obese individuals will lose a lot of weight fairly quickly while training; those with less to lose may actually find that their weight is more stable, despite their fitting into their spandex more gracefully. And remember that a person-in-training will eat more than the average individual—but you can still make good choices, even when you are eating more.

Solution #159

Dance

Dancing is the ultimate nonexerciser's exercise. Exercising can feel like work. People who exercise do things like "warm up" and "sweat" for no higher purpose than the calories burned. What fun is that? While burning calories is enough to keep some people going, many simply can't handle the concept of exercising just because they are supposed to.

This brings active pursuits like dancing to the forefront for many individuals—especially older people. Traditional ballroom styles are great for couples, and dance aerobics classes are at every gym, community center, and senior center. And unlike types of exercise that require a membership or heavy equipment, most kinds of dance aerobics can be done in the privacy of your own home with a DVD program that suits you.

Not only has research shown that dancing burns as many calories as jogging or cycling, but reality television has now "legitimized" it by broadcasting the weight loss of ordinary people week by week. Check out the Oxygen Network's *Dance Your Ass Off* at http://dyao.oxygen. com to get inspired. Dance Dance Revolution?

Solution #160

Run Barefoot

In 1970, University of Oregon track coach Bill Bowerman poured liquid urethane into a waffle iron in his garage, and running shoes have never been the same. But in our efforts to use the best technology to support our feet, we may be changing what evolution took millions of years to accomplish.

Maybe we are supposed to be running barefoot.

A recent study determined that barefoot runners tend to strike the ground mostly on the front or middle of the foot, whereas runners in cushioned shoes land on their heels—and this places much more stress on the foot. It is suspected that changing our stride in this way has led to the high prevalence of injuries in runners as compared to participants in many other recreational sports.

Does barefoot running burn more calories? The jury is still out. Most experts agree that running on the beach or on soft surfaces may require you to burn more calories, but we do not have as much information about running on harder surfaces. One argument is that if barefoot running is more efficient and results in fewer injuries, then it will make it easier for more people to be active for longer. Sounds like a good public health message, if you ask me.

Running researchers suggest that if you are going to take up barefoot running, you should transition to it slowly so that your body gets used to a new strike. And if you are concerned about acorns, rocks, or glass hurting your feet, consider a low-profile running shoe or Vibram FiveFingers to protect your tootsies.

ACT

Solution #161

Get Up, Get NEAT

NEAT, or non-exercise activity thermogenesis, is the energy we expend that is not related to sleeping, eating, or purposeful sportslike activities used to burn calories. It is the way that scientists look at the calories we unintentionally burn while brushing our teeth, tapping our feet, or walking around in circles while we talk on the phone.

The prevailing opinion seems to be that NEAT is biologically determined—i.e., some people are born to fidget. But it is also something that we can have some control over when we put our minds to it. Simple decisions made toward being more active, even when we are not exercising, can help burn calories that would otherwise go unburned.

Take standing, for example. Pretty easy, right? One study found that mildly obese individuals are sitting down for about two more hours per day than people of normal body weight. Standing without any further effort might burn an additional 350 calories per day. Depending on leisure-time activities and occupation, NEAT can vary among individuals by as much as 2,000 calories per day. That's a lot of standing.

Mayo Clinic researchers have called NEAT "the crouching tiger hidden dragon of societal weight gain." They note that the increase in obesity over the past century may reflect our increasingly sedentary lifestyle. Obviously other factors are at play, but they suggest that adopting a less sedentary "NEAT-o-type" lifestyle could help obese individuals lose weight. They also point out the need for societal changes to promote "active living."

While some researchers have looked at the introduction of exercise equipment into the workplace, the authors of one study actually examined how we might sit differently to expend some calories. They compared sitting in a traditional office chair while performing clerical work to sitting on a therapy ball and found that people burned more calories sitting on the ball, yet maintained productivity. It is this kind of thinking that can turn NEAT into a Solution for you.

So can you incorporate ways to become a leaner NEAT-o-type into your daily life? First of all, get up. Stand while you talk on the phone. Stand and socialize at get-togethers and family events instead of parking yourself on the couch and letting people come to you. Hide the television remote. Do a lap around the office each time you get another cup of coffee. Use the restroom upstairs rather than the one closest to you. Brush your teeth while standing on one foot. Sit on a rubber ball. Run on a treadmill. And film yourself and put it on YouTube.

Solution #162

Take Care of Your Own Lawn

The pride of home ownership can mean different things to different people. It can mean sitting in your breakfast nook with a cup of coffee as morning sunlight streams into the room while you do the crossword puzzle in *The New York Times,* a violin concerto whispering in the background. Or if you're me, it means crawling on the cold hardwood floor and splattering paint around as I touch up the dings my toddler made in the baseboard when he crashed his backhoe into the wall. Pride and insanity go hand in hand. And in the spring, when the snow melts, you also have to start thinking about your grass.

Take care of your own lawn. It's a tough economy anyway. You will save a few hundred bucks a year, and you will get a chance to mow down some calories at the same time as you take in some fresh air. The science supports it, and so will your spouse.

Researchers have put a scientific spin on "honey do" lists by determining the actual number of calories burned in performing common household and outdoor activities. The information was originally intended to help cardiologists decide what types of activities might be appropriate for heart patients. The end result is a scientifically developed estimate of calories burned doing common activities.

And the research supports a green thumb. A 130-pound person will burn the estimated calories per hour shown below for the outdoor activities. And keep in mind that heavier people will burn even more calories than lighter ones doing the same activity—a 200-pound person might burn 30 percent more than a 130-pound person.

Activity	Calories per Hour
Mowing lawn (self-propelled mower)	200
Mowing lawn (manual mower)	400–500
Gardening	300–500
Raking	250–300

Researchers found that mowing the lawn is associated with as much energy expenditure as aerobic exercise training. This year I bought a push mower, and I can vouch for it. Given that you are supposed to mow your lawn once a week, and fallen leaves need to be raked eventually, you are on the hook for quite a few Sundays spent outdoors, and even more calories burned off your waist. And if you have any ideas on what to do about moles, please let me know.

Solution #163
Use Trekking or Walking Poles

You might think that walking poles are useful for older people or for use in difficult terrain such as you might find in Nepal—or Oregon. While that may be true, trekking poles also provide some additional swing to your step that results in burning more calories on the hike, walk, or stroll you were already planning.

While most people perceive trekking poles as making walking easier, research demonstrates that using them actually increases your heart rate by about 16 percent and your calories burned by about 22 percent. For example, you might expect to burn an additional 100 calories after using the poles for one hour of walking. And they are safe, too. One group of researchers observed cardiac patients using walking poles during their monitored cardiac rehabilitation exercise program and found that using the poles resulted in a safe increase in exercise intensity without any ill effects.

There are many brands to choose from. While any pole is likely to do the job, there are poles specifically designed for fitness walking as compared to hiking and trekking on uneven surfaces. Some fitness walking poles that come highly recommended include the Exerstrider SE One-Piece Poles, FITTREK Nordic Walking Poles, Leki Supreme/Prestige Fitness Walking Poles, and the Exel Nordic Walker. In addition to instructions, many of these come with videos so that you can perfect your form.

And you do not have to be on a trail to use them. Walking poles can be used in your neighborhood as part of your daily walk. They may even make it seem easier to do those hills, while at the same time help you burn more calories.

Solution #164

Use Hand Weights While You Walk

If you think about it, exercising for its own sake really has not been done for all that long. In the era before desk jobs, refined sugar, and soccer carpools, activity was just part of everyday life. It was not until the 1970s that the fitness craze swept America, and it wasn't until the 1980s that people started to make it look sort of silly.

You might have your own memories of spandex, leggings, or knee-high athletic socks, but for me the 1980s were all about HeavyHands. It was a very simple idea: to incorporate light hand weights into walking to simulate the resistance exercise that makes cross-country skiers so fit. Add some red foam and some curved handles, and there you have possibly the most pervasive piece of fitness equipment of the 1980s.

HeavyHands are still on the market (www.heavyhandsfitness.com), and other brands of hand weights are available in sporting goods stores. In order to achieve the full cardiovascular benefits and burn more calories than you would by just walking, you need to *lift* the weights rather than just carry them. The idea is to exaggerate the normal movement of your arms when you walk rather than keep your arms pinned at your sides. Start by flexing your arms from a straightened position with the weights by your thighs to a 90-degree angle and then extending them back to the original position. Get more vigorous by bringing your hands level with your shoulders, or if you really want to turn some heads, raise them above your head with each step. Walking with weights works as well on the sidewalk as on a treadmill, and you will see some results after just a few weeks.

LIVE

Solution #165

Meditate

Dieting can be stressful, and this is probably one of the biggest reasons why people fall off the wagon. Too many things to think about and too many temptations are no fun and can actually cause anxiety. When you are on a diet, it is easy to lose perspective. Your short-term goal is obviously to lose some weight. And in the short term, mistakes and splurges can be so frustrating. But when you view your diet in the proper context of longer-term goals—your overall health and wellness—you realize that a bump or detour here or there doesn't really matter as long as you are moving in the right direction. The Flex Diet's mantra is that you can choose the small steps you will take to get there—if you trip every so often, it's just not that big a deal. But when you feel that things are moving too quickly for you, it's easy to forget.

So take a minute. Maybe even five. And meditate. Find some time when you can tune everything else out and close your eyes. Think about the path you are taking, and recognize that you are moving forward, even if it is more slowly than you might like or expect. Breathe deeply. Relax. Then open your eyes and press on.

Solution #166

Use a Financial Incentive to Reward Your Weight Loss

They say that money changes everything. But can it change your weight? The concept here is that money can make people do some amazing things. Take reality television, eBay, or Japanese game shows, for example. People have realized over the years that financial incentives can result in some pretty impressive displays of behavior—and it makes sense that similar incentives could theoretically impact *changes* in behavior as well.

Companies have been using financial incentives for years. Employers use bonuses to motivate employees to perform at certain levels, and even offer specific rewards related to particular accomplishments. Large insurance companies, for example, may give out a free vacation to agents who have met certain benchmarks. It is a way to keep employees happy, engaged, and ambitious, and it keeps business profitable and moving forward.

Similarly, research studies indicate that if you pay yourself per pound lost, you will lose more weight than if you do it for free. But can these results be sustained? It seems to depend on how much money you have. Once the financial incentives end, the benefits appear to diminish. However, this is similar to how incentives work with many types of behavior. It also does not seem to stray too far from general principles of weight loss—if you go back to your old habits, the weight comes back.

So how do you put incentives into your own life? Be creative. Consider setting aside a fund with an amount from each paycheck that you might normally use for fun things—like a new outfit, music downloads, or a movie. Then develop a contract with yourself (a significant other can help) where you get rewards for meeting small goals. If you continue to set aside money each month, you can keep this going. And if you gain back the weight, you have to make a deposit back into the account. Get your friends involved or talk to your company's wellness committee about creating a lottery—studies also indicate that this form of incentive works well, particularly in larger groups. This helps explain why corporate versions of *The Biggest Loser* have cropped up in workplaces everywhere. In the meantime, you will learn to integrate some lifestyle choices that you will maintain even once the well runs dry.

Solution #167

Play Active Video Games

This is my dream Solution.

Until recently, video games and weight loss were not typically mentioned in the same sentence. But the Nintendo Wii and Dance Dance Revolution have brought "exergaming" to the masses—and with the development of Wii Fit, game makers were finally making the statement that a gaming experience could actually be good for you.

When the energy expenditure related to actively playing video games is calculated, it seems that it is similar in intensity to light-to-moderate traditional physical exercise, like walking or even light jogging. In fact, one study even found that playing video games was associated with burning approximately 350 calories per hour—that's more than walking at three miles per hour. And unlike walking, it can be done at night or when it is twenty below zero outside. As might be expected, the more active games that incorporate dancing or higher-energy sports burn more calories.

One criticism of video gaming as exercise is that it needs to be done frequently and consistently in order to have any beneficial effect. This is true, but I would hazard a guess that many people's Wii or Xbox gets more time than the treadmill gathering dust in their basement. Video gaming also has some advantages of being social (if you like), and it is a nice option for seniors, who can use it in conjunction with physical therapy and to augment rehabilitation.

Solution #168

Stop Smoking Marijuana

Stop giggling.

Pretty much everyone knows, whether from personal experience, college parties, or Judd Apatow movies, that people who smoke marijuana develop a curious side effect known in medical circles as "the munchies." An increase in appetite for high-carbohydrate and high-fat snacks is a real side effect of marijuana intoxication—people don't generally *jones* for carrot and celery sticks.

So as you think about Solutions that may apply to your own life— or maybe a friend's life?—consider cutting down on your marijuana exposure. There are many other benefits which we are not going to get into, but decreasing snacking and lowering calories leads to weight loss—and that is why you are here.

Research into marijuana and body weight shows that both casual and heavy use is associated with weight gain and consuming 40 percent more calories—primarily in the form of snacks. In addition, weight gain is greater than would be predicted just by food calorie intake alone. One reason for this in the long term might be alcohol use. Frequent users tend to drink about three times the amount of alcohol as those who don't smoke pot at all. These empty calories plus a bagful of cheese puffs equal inches on your waistline that you won't care about while you are adding them on, but will regret later. The potential weight-loss benefit of quitting depends on your current level of use. Reconsider your extra-curricular activities and get high on life instead.

Solution #169

Try Acupuncture

Acupuncture is the practice of inserting very fine needles into specific points on the body for a therapeutic purpose, whereas acu*pressure* is the kinder, gentler version in which physical pressure is applied to those points. There is a lot of controversy about whether acupuncture and acupressure live up to their claims—one of the challenges is finding research like that used to evaluate traditional medicines and other inter-ventional therapies. Fans of acupuncture believe that it can help control appetite, increase the feeling of fullness, and also decrease stress, anxiety, and depression, which can lead to unhealthy eating behaviors.

Acupuncture treatment for weight reduction focuses on the ears. The fold of skin in front of the opening of the ear (the tragus) is an acupres-sure point for feeling full. Most studies of acupuncture for weight reduc-tion target this area. One study found that eight weeks of acupuncture was associated with an eight-pound weight loss. Another found that adding acupuncture to a calorie-controlled diet and fifteen minutes of walking a day was associated with an extra pound of weight loss monthly as compared to diet and walking alone. These findings have led some practitioners to recommend a procedure called ear stapling, in which staples are surgically placed in the ears to provide long-term stimulation of acupressure points. I personally do not recommend this, as I feel that the risk of infection combined with the lack of convincing data makes it too high-risk.

If needles are not your thing, studies are under way to examine the effectiveness of acupressure alone for weight loss. But don't plan to squeeze your ears yourself during meals to reduce your appetite—you need to stick with a professional. For best results, go with a doctor's recommendation for a certified acupuncturist with a good reputation in your local area. Sessions typically last an hour and may be scheduled once or twice a week. You can also find an acupuncturist through the American Association of Acupuncture and Oriental Medicine (www .aaaomonline.org) and the American Academy of Medical Acupuncture (www.medicalacupuncture.org).

Solution #170

Change Your Commute

Nobody likes to commute. Whether you live in the city and take public transportation or reside in the suburbs and fight traffic both ways, commuting always seems to feel like a waste of time. Some people take advantage of this and use their commute to get some work done on the train, and many of us read, listen to music, or watch videos to pass the time. But commuting is another opportunity to incorporate some movement into your day. And remember that your commute is not over until you arrive at your work station.

So bike to work. Get off at an earlier bus stop and walk the rest of the way. Leave your car on the top level of the parking structure and take the stairs. Park a five-minute walk away from the front door. Commit to modifying your commute to get in an extra ten minutes on your feet. Write down your plan and stick to it.

Solution #171

Get Hypnotized

Hypnosis appears to be effective for small amounts of weight loss when combined with psychotherapy. One review of twenty different studies found that adding hypnosis to behavior modification counseling is associated with an additional six to eight pounds of weight loss. It appears that hypnosis helps people better incorporate the suggestions of behavioral modification that are offered in therapy—it provides psychological reinforcement for recommendations to eat more healthfully and change behaviors. Weekly consultations for at least eight weeks are recommended, and the benefits appear to increase with longer duration of therapy.

If you do a quick survey on the Internet, you may be led to think that buying a pocket watch and a few CDs with a waterfall on the cover could be your quick ticket to a svelte figure. Not the case. The only studies of audio programs suggest that they do not result in significant weight loss. Start by talking to your doctor (rather than looking online) to find a reputable professional that you can trust. Look for a practitioner with a hypnotherapy certification (C.Ht.) and memberships in professional organizations that require specific educational standards, like the International Medical and Dental Hypnotherapy Association, the International Association of Counselors and Therapists, and the National Guild of Hypnotists.

Solution #172

Chew Gum Four Times a Day

Recent research regarding chewing gum has found that the small increase in energy expenditure related to the rhythmic "exercise" of chewing could have some ramifications for weight loss. The act of chewing gum may also reduce appetite for snacks throughout the day. Realistically, you have to be pretty inactive to have chewing gum play a significant role in your weight-loss plan. But the research is intriguing.

Chewing gum may play a role in weight loss in two different ways. The first is with respect to the actual number of calories burned by chewing the gum itself. When researchers from the Mayo Clinic measured calories burned at rest and then after chewing gum for twelve minutes, they found that calories burned per hour increased by about 20 percent. Chewing gum is similar to the difference between sitting in a chair and moving around your house. Small, but it adds up.

The other potential benefit of chewing gum is that it will keep you away from chips, pretzels, candy bars, and other high-glycemic foods that go straight to your waist. One study found that people who chew gum once an hour are less hungry for snacks, have less of a sweet tooth, and consume fewer calories at snack time than people who do not chew gum.

But chew in moderation. Regular chewing gum typically has fewer than 10 calories per stick, but they can add up. Sugar-free gum contains about 1.25 grams of sorbitol, a sweetener also used in sugar-free candies. Eating more than 20 grams daily (around fifteen sticks of gum) can cause the gum to act as a laxative, which can lead to diarrhea—which is not good for your health. So if you are interested in chewing gum to burn some extra calories and hopefully reduce snacking, limit your chewing to right after lunch and dinner, and as a snack midmorning and midafternoon when you might be having other cravings.

Solution #173

Just Watch the Movie

Let's hope you are not eating too many of your meals in movie theaters. But the food choices in movie houses have exploded in variety since you were a kid. Now you can find slushies, nachos, and hot dogs, not to mention the old standards. And movie theaters create the ultimate intentional distraction while you snack on an extra-large buttery popcorn or guzzle your thirty-second ounce of sugary soda. The good news is that there is not an intermission, so you have only one opportunity to order at the concession stand. The bad news is that you are consuming more than 1,000 calories during a seventy-nine-minute animated children's feature whose lead character is a talking mouse pad.

The best choice of all is to cut out food and beverages during movies. If you are thirsty, grab a bottle of water. If you are hungry, eat lunch or dinner beforehand. And if you are bored, the red exit lights are at either side of the screen. But if snacking is an essential part of your movie experience, consider the following. You already know that concession stand candy tends to be packaged in larger sizes than candy you might buy in a store. Despite the number of "recommended servings," you also know that you are pretty unlikely to bring an opened chocolate bar home to enjoy later. Most people will eat the whole thing and consume even more calories than if they were eating it as a normal snack. And while popcorn can certainly be a healthy snack, popcorn glowing with yellow buttery topping is most definitely not. Finally, the beverage will seal your fate as you loosen your belt during the closing credits.

Small increments in price might convince you that ordering a larger soda or popcorn is a better deal. But remember that if you get more food, you eat more food. This has actually been studied in the movie theater setting. Moviegoers who ate popcorn from large containers ate 45 percent more than when given medium-sized containers. And in a funny twist, some participants were given stale popcorn, and they still ate a third more when it was presented in a larger serving size. Given that a large popcorn can run more than 1,300 calories, this is a belly-bursting finding.

Movie Theater Food and Beverage Tips

1. Order the smallest size available.
2. Avoid anything with meat or cheese.
3. Don't have butter on the popcorn.
4. Share your candy.
5. If you buy candy, consider Mike & Ike or Gummi Bears—lower in calories and with essentially no fat.
6. Avoid chocolate- and peanut-based treats.
7. Choose water instead of a large soda and save over 300 calories.

The average person goes to about six movies a year, and younger people and older people tend to go even more frequently. If you go to the movies at least once a month, avoiding the concession stand entirely could save you at least 1,000 calories. And with the money you save, you could go twice as frequently.

Solution #174

Change Your Environment to Avoid Temptation

People continually create situations that impact their eating choices without their knowing it. If you serve your friends a buffet of nachos, chicken wings, pizza, and beer, it is guaranteed that they will stuff themselves into inebriated bliss. But if you serve that same group of friends a healthy salad, bowls of fruit, and sparkling water, they will eat much healthier . . . and you probably will never have to host a Super Bowl party again.

When given a choice, many people will choose a less-healthy alternative. But if choices are limited, or unhealthy choices are made to be less convenient, behavior can be guided toward healthier options.

Do you think you are immune to the power of convenience? Try sitting at a bar, enjoying a pint, and completely ignoring the salty, crunchy peanuts sitting beckoningly in the bowl right in front of you. Hungry? Then check out a study in which researchers examined the effect that just changing the location of a candy dish had upon the eating behavior of unsuspecting office workers. Covering a candy bowl with an opaque cover resulted in people eating two fewer pieces a day. Moving the dish off the desk—just *six feet away*—resulted in eating two fewer pieces per day. These simple changes can reduce your calorie intake every day.

This deliciously simple study illustrates the impact of your environment on what you eat and what you drink. You do not need to have a Super Bowl party or make frequent trips to bars to change your environment in a healthy way. Start at home. Do a pantry sweep at least once a month. Throw out anything that contains trans fats. Put the brownie mix and the bag of pretzels on a higher shelf. Lose the candy dish. And keep a bowl of fresh fruit front and center. Make losing weight *convenient*. Build living and work spaces that reinforce your goals and render unhealthy choices harder to make.

Solution #175

Reduce the Amount of Time You Spend Watching Television

Watching television is associated with two things. The first is food. People eat more when they watch television. The second is being overweight. Your challenge? Watch less television.

As you know, whether you enjoy TiVo, your cable company's DVR, Hulu, Apple TV, or Netflix, the way you watch television has changed significantly since you were a kid. While people continue to spend a significant amount of time in front of the television (or computer screen), we are no longer at the mercy of fixed-time programming. We watch our shows pretty much when we want to watch them. That allows some people to consume even more television, and it permits others to watch more efficiently.

Unfortunately, as television has become more convenient to watch, doing other things becomes less convenient—and those things may include reading, family time, studying, or even . . . exercise. This is not to say that if you were not watching television you would be training for a marathon. But if you are not sitting on the couch, you are doing *something*. And doing something burns more calories than doing nothing at all.

Multiple research studies have explored the relationship between television viewing and being overweight, particularly in children and adolescents—truly a captive audience. But more recent findings have emerged regarding adults and television watching, and the cable companies will not be too happy. Women who watch only one hour of television a day have a body mass index 1.8 points lower than women who watch three hours of television a day. Watching more television is associated with an almost 50 percent higher risk of being overweight or obese. Not only are television watchers generally less active, but they also consume more sweet and salty snacks as well as sugar-sweetened beverages.

Studies of television "interventions" with children have been very encouraging. One study found that reducing television time by half was associated with a significant reduction in body mass index. One might imagine that a highly motivated and more insightful adult population (the kids were not told why they were watching less TV) with greater options for physical activity and a better understanding of healthy snacking might achieve even better results.

Solution #176

Laugh for Thirty Minutes a Day

If you are trying to lose weight, sometimes you just have to laugh at yourself. Checking food labels, scarfing down fruit and almonds and water so that you can avoid that slice of pizza, going for walks instead of going for muffins, taking the stairs . . . Sometimes you need a break. There is nothing like sitting down at the end of the day and reading a funny book or blog, hanging out with family or friends, or just talking on the phone and having a laugh—and forgetting about everything else.

Did you know that laughing actually raises your metabolism? Just about 2 calories per minute—but it's something! And some researchers estimate that by increasing your heart rate by 10 to 20 percent above your baseline, laughing for just fifteen minutes can burn an extra 10 to 40 calories. That means if you laugh for thirty hours straight, you will lose a pound. We're talking serious results. Weight loss is about sacrifice—you know what you need to do.

If you have reached this point and suspect that this Solution is a joke, you may be right. But do me a favor and tack this one on in addition to the rest of the Solutions you've already chosen. It may not help you lose a significant amount of weight, but laughter is, after all, the best medicine.

Solution #177

Wait Twenty Minutes Before Eating Snacks or Eating Dessert

Take some time. Snap decisions to grab a handful of pretzels or order a slice of cheesecake occur all the time, and they happen without planning and even without hunger. Wait twenty minutes before spontaneously snacking to make it *less* spontaneous. And if you wait twenty minutes before considering dessert, chances are you will not want it anymore. The problem with random snacks is that they do not tend to decrease the number of calories we consume later in the day. Research has shown that eating high-carbohydrate snacks will not make a difference in what you eat for dinner. We know that spontaneous eating is not typically "counted" in our internal food diary, and we do not tend to cut back later to compensate. So wait twenty minutes to allow yourself to reconsider. Chances are, you will.

Solution #178

Use Blue

Blue is an inherently unappetizing color. Imagine eating blue rice, a blue sandwich, or blue gravy. The reason for this is not entirely certain, but it is probably not a coincidence that blue is not a color that occurs naturally in many foods.

It is well known in the restaurant industry that colors like red and yellow stimulate the appetite—many restaurants incorporate this into their décor and advertising. This is interesting when you consider that McDonald's, Burger King, Pizza Hut, and KFC all use red as the primary color in their logos.

If you want to get creative, consider painting your kitchen or dining room blue. It will not help with resale, but it may impact your subconscious. And if you do not want to be so extreme, buy some blue plates and bowls to achieve a similar effect. And there is always food coloring.

Solution #179

Brighten Your Environment

Seasonal affective disorder is well known to people who live at northern latitudes. The idea that less ambient daylight is associated with depressed mood and decreased motivation has been well researched. But most people do not realize that less light is also associated with a higher risk of obesity.

It is often assumed that obesity is more prevalent in colder climates because the weather makes outdoor pursuits less inviting. Also, when you wear a parka rather than a bathing suit or a tank top, you may be less concerned about how you look. But research suggests that the amount of ambient light itself plays a significant role. Rates of obesity differ depending on exposure to sunlight, even in areas with similar climates. This has led some to think that bright light may actually be a bright idea to reduce appetite and help with weight loss.

Light therapy has been used previously for people with significant seasonal affective disorder as well as nonseasonal depression. Bright-light interventions for appetite were first used to treat binge-eating episodes in people with eating disorders. And newer research suggests that a bright-light intervention may reduce the risk of obesity and can actually change eating patterns in overweight and obese individuals.

Exposure to bright light for just one hour each day has been associated with significant reduction in body fat. Bright light has been shown to increase serotonin levels, which may play a role in carbohydrate metabolism. Higher serotonin levels may also reduce overall fat intake. Finally, brighter light motivates activity, and generally improves outlook—both of which impact lifestyle choices related to becoming overweight.

While we would all like to weekend in the Bahamas, you can brighten up your environment at home at a lower cost. Open the blinds and install brighter bulbs, especially in places where you cook, eat, and exercise. Consider buying a light box and keep it on while you read, exercise, or clean a room. There are many types available online; you can get ideas at websites like www.naturebright.com and www.sunbox.com.

Solution #180

Listen to Music While You Exercise

Music sets the tone. You can be easily motivated, depressed, or annoyed by what you listen to on your iPod or stereo. As many people have discovered, listening to music can make exercise less monotonous and more fun. It can inspire them while they're trying to get up that hill or just around the block. And scientists have tried to determine whether it can make exercise more efficient.

Research shows that people who consistently listen to music while exercising are more likely to adhere to a regular exercise program. Music also tends to make us move more quickly and exercise for longer durations, and thus burn extra calories.

Even when intensity and time are held constant, exercise appears to become more efficient with music in the background. In one study of men and women working out on treadmills, the participants were asked to do the same workout with no music, slow music, and fast music. The results? Fast music burned an extra 40 calories an hour.

Songs that have 120 to 140 beats per minute appear to be the best for bringing up your heart rate and your motivation. Think "Dancing Queen" by ABBA, "Don't Stop the Music" by Rihanna, and "Know Your Enemy" by Green Day. It is better to create a mix on your iPod or buy a CD of workout music than to listen to the radio, since radio stations vary the tempo of their music. And the last thing you want is a commercial break.

Solution #181

Brush Your Teeth After Meals

Most people brush their teeth in the morning and before bed, despite their dentist's recommendation to brush after every meal. Brushing after meals improves your dental hygiene by removing food particles from your mouth; this decreases bacteria, reduces plaque, and brings down the risk of tooth and gum disease. If that isn't enough to make you change your habits, then maybe this will: brushing your teeth and using minty toothpaste can make sweet desserts and snacks seem less appetizing.

Have you ever had a glass of orange juice soon after brushing your teeth? Pretty awful, right? This is probably thanks to sodium lauryl sulfate, a compound used in toothpaste to create the sudsy sensation that makes your mouth feel clean. Sodium lauryl sulfate has the added effect of suppressing your tongue's sweet receptors and making its bitter receptors more sensitive. The end result? Sweet things taste bitter.

Use this to your advantage by brushing your teeth shortly after eating. You will be less likely to crave sweet desserts or snacks. Some people like to use breath strips or breath mints to achieve a similar effect. But toothpaste not only may work better than these, but it also helps to keep your teeth clean.

Solution #182

Turn Off the Food Channel

People obsess about television cooking programs, chef competitions, and forays into the weird, wild, and wonderful world of food. And after you spend a half hour being tempted by *America's Best Barbecue* or *Cookie Wars,* jumping on the treadmill is pretty much the last thing you want to do. Being entertained by food makes you crave it.

Advertisements do not help either. Television commercials are strategically placed to impact the behavior of the people watching them. If you watch football, you are going to be tempted to have a beer or buy a truck. If you watch Saturday morning cartoons, you will want a new toy. And if you enjoy afternoon talk shows or food programming, you are probably going to want to have a snack.

Parents have long realized that companies are marketing directly to their children, but often they do not realize that even seemingly harmless television advertisements during their own programming influence their behavior. Research shows that food advertising that promotes even the nutritious aspects of food (as opposed to the taste) will result in increased consumption of both healthy and unhealthy snacks.

So if a fifteen-second commercial can impact your diet, then imagine what an hour-long program called "Pizza, Burgers, and Steak" could do. Change the channel.

Solution #183

Buy a Headset

In the old days, people were tethered to their telephone by an extension cord. Now, cordless and cell phones are the norm, and your movements are not as limited. But consider getting a headset for your cordless or cell phone so that you can really move around, completely hands free. It will motivate you to walk around the house or do household chores while you talk instead of sitting in one place. Many states already require you to use one in your car, so make the investment now.

Solution #184

Say No to Samples

Free food is everywhere, and it has a way of sneaking into our stomachs and tricking us into buying more. Think cheese samples or hummus at your local grocery store. Hot apple cider or cocoa at the market. Mini-meatballs at Costco or Sam's Club. And while free food rarely is served as a main course, restaurants and bars entice us with peanuts, pretzels, chips, and, of course, the breadbasket.

Maybe because it is free, or maybe just because of the relatively small portions, we tend not to include free food in our mental food diary and therefore do not make adjustments later in our total calorie consumption. But these calories count just as much as the ones we eat later on—and they tend to be salty, high in fat, and high in carbohydrates. So say no to samples. Detour the dip. Pass by the pigs in a blanket. Free food is not really free.

Solution #185

Bring Your Own Airplane Snacks

Airline travel is not what it used to be. While we used to complain about how bad airline food was, now we are complaining that we do not get enough of it. So each time you fly, you are setting yourself up for a few hours of probable boredom without a decent meal. Airlines have responded to the demand by selling snacks in addition to the strangely spiced nut mix and packaged "biscuits" you get with your drink. Add this to the deep-fried pretzel you had in the terminal or the candy bar you brought on board, and you are in for a high-calorie, low-nutrition flight.

Bring your own snacks for the flight and stay in control. Parents of young kids are experts at this; they produce bags of goldfish crackers and pretzels from seemingly bottomless diaper bags. You can do the same, but instead of bringing salty, high-carbohydrate treats, think dried fruits or fresh vegetables. Bags of mini-carrots or edamame will keep you full from New York to Chicago, and if you separate your snacks into several servings, you will find yourself pressing the call button less frequently.

If you really want to impress the person sitting next to you, bring along some dried cherries for a healthy snack. In addition to their natural antioxidant and anti-inflammatory properties, cherries contain melatonin, which helps regulate our circadian rhythms and biological clock. Eating a handful of cherries before settling in on your next trans-continental flight will keep you full and might even fight your jet lag the following day.

Solution #186

Set the Alarm on Your Computer

Time passes quickly when you are sitting at your computer, whether you are surfing the Internet, playing World of Warcraft, or finishing up work after you have put the kids to bed. Hours can pass by before you know it. So set the alarm on your computer to go off every hour or every half hour. It will remind you to get up and move around your house or office—take at least a five-minute active break each hour. Not only will you be burning some calories, but your neck and eyes will thank you too. Similarly, you can set the alarm on your mobile phone to do the same—placing it on vibrate will avoid interrupting others while reminding you to get on your feet.

Solution #187

Give Your Seat to Someone Else

Some people are stuck with a daily commute. And even if you are getting off a stop early to get a little walking in before you get to work or you have taken the leap to riding your bicycle instead, there are still plenty of times when you find yourself on the subway, commuter train, or bus. Believe it or not, that is a hidden opportunity to burn some calories.

Stand up. Give your seat to someone else. Not only will you win points in the politeness department, but you will raise your metabolism by stretching your legs. As we noted earlier, research shows that skinnier people spend more of their day standing than overweight people. So take the opportunity to get on your feet while taking public transportation.

And if you really want to burn some calories, there are some easy (and not terribly obvious) exercises you can do to help tone your core muscles or your legs in the process. Tighten your stomach and butt for five seconds, and then relax for five seconds. Stand with your feet together and do calf raises—mix slow, medium, and fast speeds and try it on one foot to challenge yourself. Stand with your feet at shoulder width and slowly lift one foot a few inches off the floor. Try maintaining your footing without holding on to a bar or strap, but keep it within an easy reach just in case you need it! Or else someone might be giving up a seat for you.

Solution #188

Kiss Your Partner Ten Times a Day

It is hard to find scientific data that details the number of calories people burn during intimate activity, but in the end . . . does it really matter? While you probably are not thinking about intimacy as a way to lose weight, it may make losing weight more fun. Some people who are overweight or obese avoid intimacy—this doesn't mean just sexual activity; it can include holding hands, hugging, or kissing. But as people lose weight, they need to overcome some barriers that they may have imposed previously.

Intimacy therapy has actually been shown to be beneficial in people who are trying to lose a significant amount of weight. Intimacy is validating and reinforces the choices you are making—it means that your partner is there with you, supporting you along the way. And if being more intimate is on your mind, it may subtly impact some of the choices you are making, from giving just a little more effort in the weight room to maybe putting down the second beer or piece of chocolate cake. And, yes, it burns calories too!

Solution #189

Don't Order Room Service

Room service is the epitome of convenience. There is nothing quite like settling into your hotel room for the night in an unfamiliar city, when a knock comes on the door—your cheeseburger is here. Let's face it, convenience is the unspoken enemy of dieters everywhere. Easy decisions are often the ones you want to avoid, like getting candy bars from vending machines, a milkshake in the drive-through, and of course, room service at a hotel. Not only are you ordering food in your room rather than taking those extra steps down to the lobby, or even exploring the neighborhood and taking a walk after you eat, but people rarely make the healthiest dining choices from the confines of their hotel room. Even though better choices are usually available, it is the burgers, Caesar salads, and pizza that eventually make their way onto the tray. Get out of your room, see the sights, and find something *good* to eat.

Solution #190
There's an App for That

Many of us are sporting an iPhone these days. And while other smartphones offer calculators, cameras, and e-mail services, the iPhone's clearest advantage has always been the apps. Applications are programs that you can download wirelessly to your telephone. At last count there were more than fifty thousand, the majority of which are free or cost two dollars or less. As you might expect, there are huge numbers of applications that target fitness, diet, and weight loss. A swipe of your finger on the screen can give you incredible amounts of information that will help you learn more about nutrition, counting calories, recording activity, and even counting steps. Having the information so close at hand may make you more likely to use it. These apps will get you started.

APP	COST	WHAT IT DOES
GymGoal ABC	Free	Teaches you 280 gym exercises with animations.
GoodFoodNearYou	Free	Recommends nearby healthy food options based upon your GPS location.
MiMeals	$0.99	Helps you plan out your meals for the week, stores recipes, and keeps a grocery list.
iFitness	$1.99	Twelve fitness routines, some of which are tailored toward specific needs (e.g., business travel, body toning for women, exercising at home).

APP	COST	WHAT IT DOES
iTreadmill	$2.99	Uses a pedometer to help you track speed, distance, steps, and calories.
iBody	$9.99	Records and tracks your progress.
FitnessBuilder	$19.99	Offers an extensive library of tailored fitness routines and a tool to help you build your own routines.

Solution #191

Clean Out Your Closet

Retail therapy should be a part of every diet. This is because clothing can be a significant motivator if you wear it right. Good behaviors are reinforced when you feel good about how you look in clothes. And just because you may still be trying to lose weight, this does not mean that you can't look great in clothing that fits you well.

It is time to finally clean out your closet and set aside clothing that doesn't fit. This is more than a quick scan through your wardrobe to see what you like and don't like—it is a calorie-burning, standing-in-front-of-the-mirror investment that you should devote some time to early on in your diet.

The first step is to make three piles. The first pile should include the things that fit you well today. Hang these back up or put them back in your dresser where they belong. When you are preparing to get dressed for the day, it is discouraging to find things that look lousy or feel too tight. While keeping a favorite dress or pair of pants nearby can be a motivator, staring down a dozen size 4 skirts from college can be pretty disheartening and will send you straight toward a bowl of ice cream.

The second pile should include those size 4 skirts, skinny jeans, and business suits that you haven't worn in a while. Keep them because you will be wanting them later on, but store them out of sight. You already know that you are trying to lose weight—you don't need your jeans snickering in the background.

Finally, the third pile should include anything that is more than a size bigger than you are today. It is encouraging to know that, yes, there are clothes that are bigger than you are, which means that you have already started moving things in the right direction. But keeping those clothes on hand gives you an excuse to wear them—and baggy sweatshirts and drawstring pants invite snacks, and baggy suits just look sort of silly. Get rid of them.

Now that you have made space in your closet, it is time to go shopping. Get inspired by clothing you want to wear—it is okay to buy a pair of pants one size too small once in a while, but try to focus on good fit. Bring along your spouse or a friend (okay, maybe just a friend) who will be honest. Ask the salesperson's opinion. Get a few basics that will leave you feeling confident, inspired, and motivated to keep going in the right direction. Make a mental note of some items that you like but that do not fit perfectly right now—and set some goals. When you reach them, you can splurge.

Solution #192

Start a Garden

Gardening is a holistic weight-loss activity that will benefit you literally from soil to stomach. Research shows that you can burn between 200 and 300 calories an hour while you dig, plant, weed, and pick. You will improve your flexibility and strength while getting some fresh air and feeling productive. And you will not want all that hard work to go to waste. Garden vegetables are some of the healthiest foods—great sources of fiber and vitamins with essentially no fat and few simple carbohydrates. Commit yourself during this growing season to a real working garden, one that will let you pick vegetables for cooking and snacks every week. So while you burn calories, you will be saving money too.

Solution #193

Make Social Outings Active Rather Than Food Oriented

We know that meals eaten in restaurants tend to be higher in calories, fat, and, salt than meals we prepare at home. And we also know that when we get together with friends we are more likely to drink more alcohol, get dessert, and have multiple courses—this occurs whether we are eating out or having a dinner party or potluck at home. It turns out that when food is integral to a social gathering, we consume more calories.

The Solution is not to stay at home, but rather to make time with friends oriented more toward activities than toward food. Plan a trip to a bowling alley, museum, or sporting event rather than a bar or restaurant. Hear live music. See a play or movie. Try to center your quality time on something other than food. While some dinner parties and restaurant events are inevitable, the idea here is to explore other options that will help you avoid taking in those extra calories.

Solution #194

Lobby to Get Menu Calorie Labeling in Your Area

In 2008, the New York City Board of Health began requiring restaurants with more than fifteen locations to clearly post calorie data about every item on the menu. The rationale was that if people realized that a large white chocolate mocha had four times the calories of a small latte, they might make different choices. We already know that about half of the people who read nutrition labels on groceries change their purchasing behavior before they leave the store. And given the number of people who go to fast-food restaurants every day (one in four Americans), the potential benefit is amazing. Researchers speculate that if restaurant customers change their behavior in response to calorie information—taking in just 100 fewer calories per meal—this change could reduce our obesity problem by about 40 percent.

Early surveys have found that 82 percent of consumers are surprised by the calorie information on the foods they normally eat—and this is starting to impact food choices as well as restaurant choices (which may be the greater benefit). Seventy-one percent of respondents are looking for lower-calorie choices, and about half are no longer ordering items that they previously enjoyed.

An interesting by-product of this change (which is making its way to other large cities) is that some restaurant chains have placed new offerings on their menus or made changes in older ones to lower calories. For example, Wendy's began putting low-calorie mayonnaise on its chicken club sandwich to lower the calories by about 20 percent—although the company stated that calorie labeling had nothing to do with the move! Starbucks, Così, and other chains have made other "coincidental" changes to their menus.

When you consider the impact that this sort of change is having on unsuspecting consumers (many of whom are not actively trying to eat healthier), you can imagine what a difference it can make for people who are trying to lose weight. Calorie labeling will help you make better choices that will save calories at the point of purchase, and will also keep you mindful of other choices you make throughout the day. More than twenty states and localities are considering similar policies, and at least four have enacted them. Take the lead in your area to make this happen. You can learn more about how to implement a menu calorie labeling policy locally by sending an e-mail to the Center for Science in the Public Interest at nutritionpolicy@cspinet.org.

Solution #195

Use Chopsticks

Chopsticks carry an obvious potential advantage for Westerners trying to lose weight: we just aren't that good at using them! Aside from the occasional visit to a Chinese restaurant, we are more accustomed to shoveling food into our mouths just as fast as we want. Herein lies the Solution.

It takes some time for your stomach to signal to your brain that you are not hungry anymore. But if you eat beyond your needs before that signal is given, the signal doesn't matter. That is why eating more slowly can be an effective way to limit your calorie intake. When thinking consciously about it is not enough, chopsticks are a sneaky way to accomplish the same thing.

One observational study found that normal-weight individuals were three times more likely to use chopsticks at a Chinese restaurant than obese people. While this doesn't prove that using chopsticks made those people thin, it does support the idea that people at lower weights may consciously or subconsciously act in ways that make overeating harder to do.

Try using chopsticks to eat your dinner at home a few nights a week. It will require you to cut your food into small pieces before you eat it, and you will spend more time working for each bite. But you may find that the food tastes better when you take the opportunity to actually enjoy each mouthful.

Solution #196

Photograph Your Food

Keeping a food diary is a very effective weight-loss tool because it allows you to reflect on what you have eaten over the course of a day as well as identify trends and patterns that you can change. But it may be even more effective to document your diet in color.

A picture is worth a thousand words, right? Take a minute to check out the website www.thisiswhyyourefat.com to see what I mean. Photos do not have people's selective memory. Photos do not forget about that dollop of sour cream or misjudge portion sizes. Photos keep us honest. And that is why photographing your food puts your diet into focus. Researchers have found that a photo food diary kept for just one week was even more effective than a traditional food diary in encouraging people to change their eating habits. Having that short pause to take the picture also gives you the opportunity to change your behavior. And the photo is a pretty graphic reminder of any mistakes. And besides, it's easier now than ever—your cell phone is with you everywhere you go.

Photograph everything you eat for one week, and then take some time to scroll through the photos. Look carefully at portion sizes, and see if you can associate certain times of day or more stressful times of the week with food choices you might make differently next time.

Solution #197

Those Shoes Are Made for Walking

Do not give yourself an excuse to be inactive. High heels, tight-fitting dress shoes, or uncomfortable clothing can be a setback when they keep you from doing what you need to do to burn calories. Think about the number of times that you have decided to take a taxi, jump on the subway, or cut your stroll short because of pinched toes, painful heels, or just feeling hot and sweaty. Nice clothes definitely have their place, but do not let them get in the way of staying on your feet.

Solution #198

See Yourself Thin

After learning about so many different ways to lose weight and become healthier, it comes down to attitude in the end. You are armed with more information than many doctors have about small changes you can make to seriously impact your weight and your life. But all the information in the world does not mean a thing if it doesn't translate into action. There is willpower, and then there is confidence. It comes down to self-perception. It comes down to believing that you can do it.

If you have spent much of your life battling extra pounds, it can be hard to stay motivated. Being slim becomes something that other people get to enjoy and experience. After a while, being overweight becomes part of your identity, and that is hard to change. But attitude and behavior are closely tied together. There is a concept in psychology called cognitive dissonance that explains this relationship. The idea is that if you want to change how you think about something, changing your behavior *first* will ultimately result in a change in attitude. Your mind needs consistency. One example of this process might be to have a longtime smoker participate in a lobbying program for antitobacco legislation or against smoking in public places. These activities would likely impact attitudes about smoking, and might actually help the person stop.

Cognitive dissonance can also work the other way. Changing your attitude should result in an appropriate change in behavior. Applying this concept to wellness and weight loss, it seems that in order to change what we do, we have to make sure that our attitude, self-perception, and confidence are there to provide support. If being healthy or thinner is a change you can actually believe in, then you just might start following the Solutions explored throughout this program.

One approach to this is to visualize your goal. Take some time to really think about the person you are trying to become and how your life might be a little bit different by picturing yourself at your weight-loss goal. You can obviously do this in your mind, but you can also have some fun with a little augmented reality. Websites like www.weightview. com (free), www.mvm.com (My Virtual Model, also free), and Weight Loss Pose (ten to twenty dollars) will help you modify your own photos or even design avatars of yourself that allow you to try new outfits on at your lower weight. There are certainly no guarantees that Photoshopping will improve your grocery shopping, but it's a fun motivator and you can print out the results and keep them on your bathroom mirror or on your cell phone. Seeing it is part of believing it.

Solution #199

Fill In the Blank

Enough about me. The Flex Diet provides 200 time-tested, evidence-based, experience-driven, and out-of-the-box Solutions to help you lose weight. But I don't have all the answers. It's your turn now. Come up with one Solution. It could be a substitution, a recipe, a way to automate your meals, or even just a mantra that helps you make better decisions. Write it down here, and follow it.

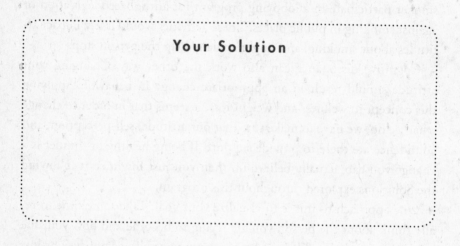

Your Solution

Solution #200

Count Your Blessings

After learning two hundred Solutions to help you lose weight and live a healthier life, you have realized that the Flex Diet is about more than just what you Eat, what you Drink, how you Exercise, how you Act, and how you Live. Wellness is about how you feel. You can be mindful, knowledgeable, and motivated to succeed, but how you *Feel* is the cornerstone of the entire program. If you don't feel good about yourself and what you are doing, the rest loses much of its meaning.

Strengthening positive emotions is a lifelong challenge for many. This has become a popular topic of research in recent years, and we have learned that not only does positive reinforcement work, but reinforcing the positive does as well. Let me explain. One study asked young adults to keep a "gratitude journal." During nearly three months, young women and men recorded five things that had happened during the previous week that made them thankful. That's it. The results? Not only did they become significantly happier and more optimistic, but they got sick less and exercised more. And their friends found them more helpful and emotionally supportive.

It's an amazingly simple concept. Giving thanks and reinforcing the positive in your life will come back to you by making you feel more positive and more motivated. Take five minutes each week and be thankful. Thankful for the people that support you. Thankful for the choices you have made. Thankful for your health and the things that make you happy. This truly is the Solution.

5

IF YOU ARE NOT PART OF THE SOLUTION, YOU ARE PART OF THE PROBLEM

You won't find a solution by saying there is no problem.

— WILLIAM ROTSLER

If you think about it, your body is not really meant to lose weight. Turn back your evolutionary clock for a minute and take a second to remember when you were living in a cave and living from meal to meal. Your body was designed for its environment—you craved salt, sugar, and fat, and you burned calories quickly because you were hunting for food and running away from saber-toothed tigers. You did not have time to gain weight, and you did not have to think about losing it. Millions of years later, your body tells you to eat the way you always did, but now you sit at a desk, watch television, and wish your Facebook status updates were about something other than sitting at a desk and watching television.

As everybody knows, obesity has skyrocketed over the past thirty years, even though we know more than ever about nutrition, and opportunities for exercise are everywhere. The statistics are truly jarring, although perhaps unsurprising to anyone who frequents shopping malls, fast-food restaurants, or much of the United States.

According to the American Heart Association, more than nine million American children and teenagers are overweight. That's *one out of six kids*. And over 70 percent of overweight adolescents will go on to become the next generation of overweight adults. Welcome to the club—there are already 142 million members. Even just twenty years ago, none of the fifty states had an obesity prevalence greater than 15 percent. But by 2007, only Colorado could claim that *less than 20 percent* of its population was obese.

It is reminiscent of that first day of law school immortalized in *The Paper Chase,* when the eminent professor says to the incoming class, "Look to your left and look to your right, because one of you won't be here by the end of the year." But many Americans would be better off these days if someone told us, "Look to your left and look to your right. Now take a good look in the mirror."

No one can debate that we are getting fatter. And when America sneezes, the world catches a cold—or at least eats Big Macs. As the world becomes further developed and Western nations become even more urbanized, diets change and lifestyles become more sedentary. As a result, obesity rates have tripled in the United Kingdom, Eastern Europe, the Middle East, and Australia since the 1980s. No wonder heart disease has beat out infections as the major cause of morbidity and mortality throughout the first, second, and third worlds.

Some people would argue that the recent catchphrase "the obesity epidemic" sensationalizes the issue and stigmatizes the overweight. The backlash has led to the fat-acceptance movement, whose supporters fight against discrimination. But another trend is the celebration of "health at every size." Some believe that the health risks of being overweight or obese have been exaggerated and are used as a cover for underlying prejudice and as an excuse to stigmatize obese people in the workplace and in social situations. Simultaneously, there is an ever-growing and well-justified frustration with what many consider to be unrealistic depictions of beauty in fashion magazines and other media. Few people are destined to be a size 2, and more people are highlighting the beauty of "real" people at higher weights. But an important distinction needs to be made between beauty and health. The risks of being overweight should not be exaggerated, but they also can't be minimized for the sake of political correctness.

SPARE TIRE VS. JUNK IN THE TRUNK

If only it were just the pounds that mattered. But you also have to think about where you are hiding them. No matter what your type, being overweight is associated with health risks. And abdominal obesity (think belly fat) appears to be associated with even worse medical outcomes, particularly when it comes to heart disease. Call it a syndrome. Call it a disease. Or just call it a terrible coincidence. The metabolic syndrome takes the worst of our risk factors for heart disease, combines them, and produces more heart attacks and strokes than you can shake an aspirin at. Abdominal obesity is one of the contributing factors in metabolic syndrome, and exercise combined with diet and lifestyle changes will not only reduce your risk of developing the syndrome, but will also likely address the abnormalities in cholesterol, blood pressure, and blood sugar that contribute to it.

Many people (and some diet books) focus on belly fat for this reason. But there is a common misconception that certain types of diets,

> ### The Metabolic Syndrome
> *(Three out of five makes the diagnosis.)*
>
> ☐ **Increased waist circumference**
> Men: greater than or equal to forty inches
> Women: greater than or equal to thirty-five inches
>
> ☐ **Elevated triglycerides**
> Greater than or equal to 150 mg/dL
>
> ☐ **Reduced HDL cholesterol**
> Men: less than 40 mg/dL
> Women: less than 50 mg/dL
>
> ☐ **Elevated blood pressure**
> Greater than or equal to 130/85 mm Hg *or* use of medication for hypertension
>
> ☐ **Elevated fasting glucose**
> Greater than or equal to 100 mg/dL *or* use of medication for hyperglycemia

or even exercises, will target belly fat specifically and lower your risk of metabolic syndrome. In reality, diet and exercise will help you reduce fat and lose weight everywhere—you may *notice* it first in your belly because that is where people tend to have the most of it. Exercises geared toward reducing belly fat (like sit-ups or crunches) may improve the tone of your abs, but you are never going to be able to show them off unless you lose weight overall.

Even though I am a cardiologist, I still find the focus on metabolic syndrome in the context of competing health risks somewhat distracting. The health risks of being overweight or obese—no matter how you package it—are too numerous to count. There are no winners here. True, the increased risk of heart attacks and strokes is most relevant to

Medical Complications of Obesity

Abdominal hernias

Abnormal cholesterol

Abnormal menses

Acid reflux

Back pain

Breast cancer

Childbirth complications

Chronic pain

Chronic venous insufficiency

Colon cancer

Coronary disease

Deep venous thrombosis

Depression

Diabetes

End-stage kidney disease

Esophageal cancer

Fatigue

Fungal infections

Gallbladder cancer

Gout

High blood pressure

Infertility

Kidney cancer

Neural tube defects

Nonalcoholic steatohepatitis

Osteoarthritis

Pancreatitis

Prostate cancer

Restrictive lung disease

Rheumatoid arthritis

Sleep apnea

Stomach cancer

Stroke

Urinary incontinence

Uterine cancer

Weakened immune system

Wound infections

what I see every day, but even I am somewhat amazed at how excess weight is correlated with *every* kind of adverse health outcome, from acid reflux to wound infections.

BMI: JUST ANOTHER THREE-LETTER WORD?

Remember the phrase "You'll know it when you see it"? The whole diet-book industry is somewhat based upon subjectivity—it's a response to people looking in the mirror. But when doctors and public health organizations get involved, we need to establish some objective scales to understand our worsening weight problem.

Let's start with the body mass index, or BMI. The BMI is a simple measurement that we use to define the relationship between weight and height. While it certainly has its limitations, body mass index is convenient and easy to determine, and therefore lends itself to widespread use in research studies and public policy documents, and in doctors' offices everywhere.

$$\text{Body Mass Index} = \frac{\text{Weight in Kilograms}}{(\text{Height in Meters}) \times (\text{Height in Meters})}$$

Calculate your BMI by dividing your weight in kilograms by your height in meters, and then divide again by height in meters. Or on the off chance that you are an American and never figured out the metric system, you can multiply your weight in pounds by 703, divide by your height in inches, and then divide again by your height in inches.

Doctors use the following table to categorize individuals based on their body mass index.

Body Mass Index	Category
Below 18.5	Underweight
18.5–24.9	Healthy weight
25.0–29.9	Overweight
30–39.9	Obese
Over 40	Morbidly obese

Keep in mind that this classification system is most useful as a general guideline. When it is applied to an individual, there are additional considerations, including one's age and any health condition that could be contributing to a weight change in either direction. For example, body mass index should not be used for children. There is a wealth of data on the relationship between weight and height in children, and the data have been converted into growth curves that pediatricians use throughout your child's development to assess an appropriate weight. Determining a child to be obese or overweight really falls under a pediatrician's expertise, as does developing a weight-loss plan for the child. However, body mass index can help in monitoring the health of the elderly. Elderly people may lose weight as a result of poor appetite or one of a number of medical conditions. In these situations, a significant change in weight or body mass index is a marker of something of concern going on and should be discussed with a doctor.

Adults should also consider their body type when using body mass index as a tool for assessing appropriate weight. People like to refer to the "muscle weighs more than fat" adage to suggest that more muscular people may weigh more than their fatter counterparts. But a pound is a pound, and a pound of muscle weighs the same as a pound of fat. However, muscle is significantly more dense than fat, so muscular people will generally weigh more than less muscular people at baseline. This can cause muscular people to be identified as "overweight" when they really are not. Even so, if you are walking around with a BMI of over 30 and can't bend down to tie your own shoes, you should probably switch from the bench press to the treadmill anyway.

Body mass index has understandably been criticized because it is so simple. For example, one study of older men showed that as body mass index increased, the risk of dying increased as well. But interestingly, a low body mass index was also associated with some increase in risk. This might suggest the role of some disease-specific causes of death, such as cancer, that could be related to lower body mass index.

While most doctors would agree that being obese (BMI > 30) is associated with increased rates of death, there is a little less consensus about the "overweight" category. Increased death rates do not really start to spike until the BMI goes above 30. And to make it more complex, the association between body mass index and death may fade as we grow older. The optimal BMI may change as we age. It appears that being "overweight" is actually more subjective than doctors would like it to be, and should probably be considered in the context of gender, smoking status, and other medical issues. So you might be asking, "Depending on my age, does this mean that being mildly 'overweight' isn't such a bad thing? And you waited until page 233 to tell me?"

FIT *AND* FAT?

Hold your horses. Let's remember the concept that not all weight is created equal—that muscle and fat have different mass and different effects on our body composition. I can't tell you how many times a healthy-appearing, athletic individual has told me that he or she needs to lose weight because of a body mass index over 25. As we are learning, following BMI so rigidly is not necessarily the best way to use the scale, so to speak. Looking in the mirror helps, too.

Some people apply a conspiracy theory to body mass index. It is true that in 1998 the United States government changed its definition of what it means to be overweight, possibly in response to some political pressure from the World Health Organization. The new classification by body mass index ignored differences between men and women, and the cut point of 25 meant that twenty-five million more Americans woke up one day in 1998 to learn that they were now overweight. Talk about waking up on the wrong side of the bed!

Not only are body mass index definitions of "overweight" and "obese" somewhat arbitrary, but a simple number cannot differentiate between muscle and fat. The fit-or-fat debate takes a humorous turn when you consider the body mass index of top athletes culled from official team and Olympic websites. Trust me, no one is calling Shaq obese. Well, at least not where he can hear them. Even Michael Phelps has a BMI of about 24.4, according to some sources. Think how many gold medals he could have won if he were *really* in shape!

From the looks of it, being a little "overweight" may not be such a bad thing. The truth is that being fit is more important than the weight itself. This was illustrated in a study of death rates among middle-aged men as related to both body mass index and fitness. The results were seemingly paradoxical. After adjusting for age, low exercise capacity was the single most important predictor of death. And survivors were noted to have an average body mass index of about one point *higher* than those who died during the study. This was true among individuals with and without heart disease. These findings were confirmed with another study that noted that both fitness and a slightly higher BMI were associated with better outcomes. If you use body mass index too strictly, "fit" can actually appear "fat," due to the effect of higher-density muscle on the measurement.

Given the limitations of body mass index, I do not recommend that people diet toward a particular body mass index. But there are other calculators out there for people who are looking for a specific goal. For example, the ideal body weight measurement, or IBW, is based upon weight, height, and gender, and like BMI, it can be calculated easily. But there are also some limitations, especially depending upon your body frame and your age. The consensus appears to be that ideal body weight may increase a bit as we age, but it's unclear whether this is really accurate, or whether it was just decided upon by older people!

Physicians sometimes use this slightly more involved formula for ideal body weight, which also uses your height, weight, and gender, but takes it a step further by considering your body frame.

> **Men:** 106 lbs for first 5 feet + 6 lbs for each inch over 5 feet
> **Women:** 100 lbs for first 5 feet + 5 lbs for each inch over 5 feet
>
> (Small frame, - 10%, large frame, + 10%)

In my opinion, this formula is still a little challenging to use, because it requires you to choose an exact target weight, rather than a more realistic general range. I have found the following tables—for women and men—to be helpful for this reason. They provide a reasonable range for any given height and body frame, so that you can define a personal, healthy goal that is actually attainable.

HEALTHY WEIGHT RANGES: WOMEN

HEIGHT	SMALL FRAME	MEDIUM FRAME	LARGE FRAME
4' 10"	102–111	109–121	118–131
4' 11"	103–113	111–123	120–134
5' 0"	104–115	113–126	122–137
5' 1"	106–118	115–129	125–140
5' 2"	108–121	118–132	128–143
5' 3"	111–124	121–135	131–147
5' 4"	114–127	124–138	134–151
5' 5"	117–130	127–141	137–155
5' 6"	120–133	130–144	140–159
5' 7"	123–136	133–147	143–163
5' 8"	126–139	136–150	146–167
5' 9"	129–142	139–153	149–170
5' 10"	132–145	142–156	152–173
5' 11"	135–148	145–159	155–176
6' 0"	138–151	148–162	158–179

HEALTHY WEIGHT RANGES: MEN

HEIGHT	SMALL FRAME	MEDIUM FRAME	LARGE FRAME
5' 2"	128–134	131–141	138–150
5' 3"	130–136	133–143	140–153
5' 4"	132–138	135–145	142–156
5' 5"	134–140	137–148	144–160
5' 6"	136–142	139–151	146–164
5' 7"	138–145	142–154	149–168

HEIGHT	SMALL FRAME	MEDIUM FRAME	LARGE FRAME
5' 8"	140–148	145–157	152–172
5' 9"	142–151	148–160	155–176
5' 10"	144–154	151–163	158–180
5' 11"	146–157	154–166	161–184
6' 0"	149–160	157–170	164–188
6' 1"	152–164	160–174	168–192
6' 2"	155–168	164–178	172–197
6' 3"	158–172	167–182	176–202
6' 4"	162–176	171–187	181–207

So what's the takeaway? It turns out that your weight *is* just a number. And talking about weight loss in terms of body mass index, ideal body weight, or even Solutions is ultimately just a way to get you to focus on changing your lifestyle to enact healthy change. You may measure your progress in pounds, by dress sizes, or by the confidence you feel on the beach or in your workplace. But true success arises from the process itself. A skinny person who smokes and eats fast food is no healthier than a heavier person who exercises regularly and eats right. The Solutions throughout this book have been framed as small changes to help you lose weight in small steps, but the sum of your Solutions is actually greater than the number of pounds you might lose. You have changed how you live. You are healthier. You feel better.

You did it.

6.

WHEN SOLUTIONS ARE
NOT ENOUGH

Extreme remedies are very appropriate for extreme
diseases.

— HIPPOCRATES

This book presents two hundred different Solutions that you can combine and integrate into your life to lose weight and become healthier. Although these Solutions are well supported and evidence-based, remember that there is no such thing as a diet miracle. Losing weight is hard work, no matter how you simplify it or make it sound interesting. But if you have a significant problem with weight and cannot lose it by conventional means, a miracle starts to sound pretty good.

Unfortunately, the diet industry hears that call, and miracles are promised every day in the form of supplements, creams, exercise equipment, and even books. And perhaps because of the way advertisers blur the lines, people do not seem to get the right information about how medical and surgical therapies for obesity can become part of *their* solution. Just talking about obesity can be difficult enough. Stigmatization and poor understanding have led us to avoid discussing obesity treatments in our medical practices and around our dinner tables. But if they might apply to you, you deserve the right information to get you started.

THINK WELLNESS, NOT WEAKNESS

Even though I am a doctor, I think that medical specialists—including cardiologists—do a disservice to their patients by placing their problems into too many categories and breaking people down into parts. While it can be easier to understand problems when you label them, and it simplifies conditions when you separate them, we may limit our ability to evaluate the entire person if we never take a look at the whole. Sure, it makes a health care provider's job easier—a specific constellation of symptoms or signs leads to a diagnosis that then prompts us to recommend a particular treatment. But in an era when medical specialists focus on individual organ systems and leave the rest to "your primary doctor," it is easy to feel swept aside if you do not fall into the right category.

It can get especially uncomfortable when you find yourself at the intersection of lifestyle and its medical consequences. Issues of addiction and impulse control come into play, and these can bring about too much focus on blame and not enough on change. But one thing I have recognized is that when we allow ourselves to think of lifestyle-related medical conditions as legitimate and complex, they lose some of their negative connotation and can be viewed more objectively. And when the conditions are viewed more objectively, they tend to be more thoroughly researched, with the goal of developing real and evidence-based therapies to treat them.

Take smoking as an example. Our societal understanding of smoking has changed so much in the past twenty years, and our medical treatments have improved significantly. As we have recognized that nicotine addiction is an actual medical diagnosis, we have become more aggressive in our attempts to treat it. We now have several medical options that are responsible for improving the lives of literally millions of individuals. The discussion is less about "willpower" or "weakness" and more about treatment. People have truly benefited because scientists and thought leaders have changed the way we think about smoking.

Obesity medicine is catching up. While obesity is still unfortunately associated in popular culture with certain personality traits, the medical consequences have gained traction in the media, and doctors are taking obesity more seriously than ever before. Research is booming, and is responsible for the many Solutions presented throughout this book. But this chapter focuses less on the choices *you* make, and more on the treatment plan that you and your doctor can make together. There are three components: medical therapies, surgical treatments, and behavioral interventions.

MEDICAL TREATMENT OF OBESITY

It is important to review our definitions of obesity if we are going to evaluate who is appropriate for treatment. Regardless of the limitations of the body mass index calculation, medical obesity is defined as a body mass index greater than 30, and surgical treatment is generally confined to people with a body mass index greater than 40. The American College of Physicians recently issued clinical practice guidelines stating that medical therapies for obesity may be offered to those individuals who have been unable to achieve weight loss through diet and exercise alone. Seven medications are referenced: sibutramine, orlistat, phentermine, and diethylpropion, and three drugs that are not approved for obesity treatment, fluoxetine, sertraline, and buproprion. Since the publication of that report, sibutramine has been pulled off the market because of an increased risk of heart attacks and strokes in people who used the drug. Please remember that pharmacologic treatment of obesity is a decision made between you and your doctor, and should be adopted only under close medical supervision.

The straight dope on medications is that current therapies do not promote as much weight loss as many people are hoping—it is unlikely that medication will help you lose more than ten pounds in the longer term. There are also concerns that weight will be regained once medications are eventually discontinued. There are emerging therapies that are still being researched, but they may not be available for some time. But in general, medical therapy is not a long-term solution.

Sibutramine

Sibutramine limits the uptake of chemicals called neurotransmitters (like norepinephrine, serotonin, and dopamine) into nerve endings—a mechanism similar to that of many medications used to treat depression. Higher concentrations of these chemicals result in decreased food intake, and therefore weight loss. Research studies suggest that year-long treatment with sibutramine is associated with weight loss of about ten pounds. However, it can also cause small increases in blood pressure, which may account for its associated increase in cardiac risk. For this reason it was pulled off the market in October 2010.

Orlistat

Orlistat prevents pancreatic enzymes from breaking down food in your digestive tract so that it will not be absorbed. Orlistat is associated with a six-pound weight loss as compared to placebo alone. But knowing its mechanism, you will not be surprised to learn that it is also associated with varying degrees of "gastrointestinal distress" in about 15 to 30 percent of users. Vitamin supplements are also often recommended. Interestingly, addition of orlistat to sibutramine is not associated with further significant weight loss, and patients are typically prescribed one or the other.

Phentermine and Diethylpropion

These drugs function as stimulants, but because of the potential for abuse, they are only approved for use for twelve weeks or less. But phentermine was actually studied over a longer period of time, so it is unclear how beneficial it might be in a three-month time frame.

Antidepressants: Fluoxetine, Sertraline, and Buproprion

It is hard to argue that there is not a link between depression, obesity, and heart disease. We have already explored how treating depression can help with weight loss. People who are depressed may experience social isolation and seek solace in food. Depression can impact motivation to make good lifestyle choices. It makes sense that treating it can help out in other areas as well. But an interesting finding is that *some* drugs used to treat depression may in fact independently promote weight loss. Whereas some antidepressants can cause weight gain, fluoxetine and sertraline are both associated with a very modest weight loss (just a few pounds). Buproprion, used to treat depression and for assistance with smoking cessation, also has some weight-loss effect. However, these drugs are not currently recommended to treat weight loss specifically, given that higher-than-typical doses are required and long-term effects are not known at this time.

SURGICAL TREATMENT OF OBESITY

Now here is where it starts to get interesting. Despite the importance of lifestyle, diet, and exercise recommendations as well as the small added impact of medical therapy, morbid obesity is treated most successfully with bariatric surgery. Morbid obesity is generally defined as a body mass index of greater than 40, although some centers offer bariatric surgery for individuals with body mass index greater than 35 when their condition is complicated by significant weight-related illnesses such as diabetes or sleep apnea. Treatment at a center with substantial surgical experience as well as appropriate follow-up is generally recommended. And remember, liposuction is not weight-loss surgery! While it will certainly result in some weight loss, it is actually pretty insignificant compared to the impact of bariatric surgery. And besides, it does not result in improvements in diabetes or other heart disease risk factors.

Weight-loss surgery is generally divided into two categories. *Restrictive* procedures limit your caloric intake by reshaping your stomach. *Malabsorptive* procedures work by functionally shortening the small bowel, thereby limiting absorption of calories. Finally, there are some combinations of the two.

Bariatric surgery is obviously a huge decision. It requires a commitment to long-term weight loss and appropriate medical follow-up. It also requires a full understanding of the risks related to surgery and the possible side effects that may come later. These are complicated procedures, and a multidisciplinary medical-surgical team can provide you with more detailed information so that you can make the best decision. Websites like www.yourbariatricsurgeryguide.com and many others can direct you to bariatric surgery centers in your area.

INTEGRATED THERAPIES

Anyone who is seriously considering medical or surgical treatments for obesity should also look into integrative approaches to help make better lifestyle choices. Behavioral strategies have been in use for over fifty years, and they generally result in more weight loss when combined with surgical or medical solutions.

Behavioral strategies for weight loss are inherently optimistic, as they imply that behaviors are in some part responsible for being overweight, and that the behaviors can be changed to help promote weight loss. Some of the strategies are cast as Solutions throughout this book, and can include everything from increasing your social supports to planning your meals to reinforcing and rewarding healthy behaviors.

But some of these strategies are most effective when incorporated into a formal weight-loss program, which may improve results overall. One review found that behavioral therapy actually increased weight loss by about fifteen pounds over a one-year period. Self-help programs are cheaper than the large-scale commercial programs, but attending the weekly meetings may result in more weight loss in the long term. More formalized cognitive-behavioral counseling has been extensively researched, particularly in the bariatric surgery population, and has been found to be very helpful in maintaining weight loss in the longer term.

Internet-based programs are an exciting and relatively recent phenomenon, and there are research findings to support their use. Structured Internet programs directed toward behavior modification have been shown to result in weight loss of greater than five pounds more than information-only websites. Benefits of texted reminders and in-person and online support groups have been described elsewhere in this book. As the Internet evolves with social networking and more sophisticated options, this area of weight loss is bound to reach greater importance. Look for more research studies and coverage in the popular and medical press. And check out www.theflexdiet.com for references, more ideas, and maybe even some more Solutions!

7

WHAT'S *YOUR* SOLUTION?

Give a man a fish and you feed him for a day.
Teach a man to fish and you feed him for a lifetime.

—Chinese Proverb

Omega-3s aside, it turns out that this simple proverb is the key to most self-help books out there. Diet books, wellness guides, and lifestyle bloggers everywhere are basically handing you a *fish*. A fish can be a tool, a system, a program, or even a Solution. The goal is to understand it and ultimately incorporate it into your own life.

The problem is that when you close the book, turn off the radio, or switch to a different channel or website, the so-called Solution can also fade to black. Authors and experts everywhere would like to think that they have communicated so effectively that their audience forever internalizes every bit of information or strategy they have shared. But we know that this isn't really the case. Check out any mall in America, any sporting event, or any fast-food drive-through and you will see Solutions passing through one collective ear and out the other. Is this forgetfulness? Or does it just highlight the difference between giving information and actually teaching it?

Before you reach the last page and close this book, let's take a second to reflect and refocus for the long journey ahead. Keeping these ideas in mind will help you get back on track when you find yourself staring down a basket of curly fries next weekend. Let's . . . go fishing.

IT WAS YOUR IDEA IN THE FIRST PLACE

Getting healthy has to be your idea first. It's not up to your doctor, your boyfriend or girlfriend, your mom, or your spouse. It can't be a commercial, an ad campaign, or a motivational speech or book. You have to take the plunge on your own terms. If you decide you want out, that's your choice too, but make sure that you understand the consequences first.

Compare your own challenge to that of someone who is trying to quit smoking. We identify five stages of change in people who smoke, but we can easily apply them to a person going on a diet, or trying to stay on one.

STATE OF CHANGE	SMOKING	DIETING
Pre-contemplative	Not ready to quit.	"I'll have another Ding Dong, please."
Contemplative	Thinking about quitting.	"I'll read this book *after* I have another Ding Dong."
Action	Ready to quit. Interested in counseling or medications.	You are hopefully doing it right now.
Maintenance	Has quit. Needs reinforcement.	The most challenging part of all.
Relapse	May need to go through the first four stages many times before quitting forever.	"I'll have another Ding Dong, please."

I have found when trying to help smokers quit that many are in the Pre-contemplative stage, and it is pretty hard to make an impact. One of the tricky aspects of dieting is that many people are *still* in the

Pre-contemplative or Contemplative stage by the time they get to the end of the book. They have the information, but are still not ready to use it. In the end, statistics and Solutions do not mean a thing if losing weight isn't *your* idea first. Make the commitment to no one but yourself. If you get into a rough spot later on, make it *your* idea to get back with the program. Looking for direction? Then find your problem first.

FIND YOUR PROBLEM FIRST

It is an easy mistake to make. People are constantly looking for a how-to before they have figured out a to-what. Easy ways to make money. Techniques for talking to attractive women or men. Methods for increasing your number of followers on Twitter. It is as if we have gotten so focused on how to beat the system, we have forgotten what we are trying to achieve. We get it in our heads that we have to keep moving. But if you don't know what you are trying to move toward, you just end up treading water. So find your problem first, and *then* you can worry about the Solution.

When it comes to a healthy lifestyle, start by thinking about a problem that you want to solve. A dress size. A bathing suit. A class reunion. A heart attack. Use that problem to motivate you, to drive you toward Solutions that will get you where you want to be. Steer yourself toward concrete goals—because concrete goals require specific measures to achieve them. The goal can be a number, like cholesterol level, blood pressure, or weight. It can be a physical goal, like doing a triathlon or even getting around the block without being short of breath. Mental and emotional goals are more elusive, but they work too. Find your problem, and *then* find your Solution.

LOOK UP

Once you have figured out your goals, it is time to put together your Solutions. That's what this book was for. You hopefully have started to incorporate dozens of different concepts presented throughout this program that will help generate a healthier lifestyle, but now it is time to commit to a longer-term path. One of the challenges people face is how to continue motivating themselves when they have already achieved their goals. Once you achieve a desired weight, it is easy to then fall off the wagon because you think you can just do it again. But this leads to a behavioral cycle in which your system "doesn't work" or you can't get back into a healthy mind-set—some people call it yo-yo dieting. It is known to be less healthy and ultimately results in a higher weight than before you started.

Follow the example of successful CEOs and other leaders in their fields. When they achieve a certain level of success, they go back to the boardroom or the laboratory or the gym and get started on a new goal. Michael Phelps is back in the pool. Apple is coming out with a better iPhone. Scientists are looking for a new cure. Their goals are moving targets. The most successful people in the world approach their own lives like entrepreneurs—they are constantly ambitious. This does not mean dissatisfied. But it does mean that when they reach one summit, they enjoy the view while at the same time planning the next expedition. *They are always looking up.*

It's time to get to work on your own personal start-up. Shave a few seconds off your personal best. Try to get off that blood pressure medicine. Plan an active vacation. Use your newfound confidence to excel in other areas of your life. Move your own target, and create your own path to reach it. It is time to make your own Solutions.

NOW GO FISH

Creating your own Solutions is easier than you might think. I ask my patients to try it every day. If you passed this one up when it was presented as Solution # 199 (page 224), take a second look. It starts with thinking about how you live your life from the time you wake up to when you go to bed, and everything in between. I have my patients keep a complete food and activity diary for at least one week—I hope you are already doing this. If you find yourself getting lost, a diary is the best way to refocus your efforts. Every glass of water, every walk around the block. Hours of sleep, minutes of treadmill, and second servings too.

Simple information can produce amazing insights. And now you have an educated filter you can use to analyze this raw data to recognize patterns and inefficiencies and ways you can change them. Approach your life like a scientist, or like a CEO—find the ways that you can become more efficient and profit from your own good choices.

The goal of this program is to personalize wellness, but the truth is that no program can work for absolutely everyone. You are an individual, and despite my best efforts, there are potential Solutions for you that I haven't thought of yet. So it is your turn to help me out, and help out others like you. I want to know *your* Solutions.

Take some time and take a look at yourself, and see if you can come up with at least one Solution that you can use to optimize your nutrition, cut out unhealthy calories, and increase your activity, exercise, and motivation. Then get online and share it. Become involved in the community. Respond to blog posts. Answer questions on Twitter. Experience is the simplest and truest path to expertise.

Share your Solutions with me by writing on the Flex Diet's wall on Facebook. They will be shared with the rest of the community, and if we get enough support, they could be the underpinnings of a new collection of Solutions compiled by readers just like you. Think of it as learning how to fish, and teaching someone else.

WELLNESS IS A VERB

While I was in college, I read a book called *Lila,* written by Robert Pirsig. Part novel and part philosophy text, *Lila* explores morality, purpose, and human relationships. One concept from the book that has stuck with me after nearly twenty years is an idea stated in the conclusion:

"Good is a verb."

The first time I read that sentence, something didn't feel right. We typically think of "good" as a quality, not an action. It may define who we are or who we are not. It may stand for a group that we want to belong to, and sometimes exclude our enemies from. But using "good" as a passive descriptor takes something out of the equation: choice. When we think about goodness as a verb and as an action, our choices can change who we are and where we belong. Good is a process. *Good is a journey.*

I ultimately found myself in medical school and specialty training, spending a lot of time with people who are often categorized according to a different system: wellness and disease. Doctors and patients judge themselves and others by this simple metric all too frequently. And we know that illness—or even just being overweight—can put us in a less desirable place, populated by individuals with less self-confidence, more symptoms, and even a need for medication. Nobody wants to be ill. And nobody wants to be part of the group of people who experience illness.

But I have learned that this way of thinking about health and disease, or wellness and illness, is an oversimplification, because it implies that our health status defines who we are. Categories take away the element of choice. Obviously, no one chooses to be sick. Genetics and environment conspire to create illness—or even a spare tire—in people with the best of intentions. But we can't ignore the impact, whether positive or negative, of the lifestyle choices we make every day on our health. Sure, there are genetics and bad luck, but there is also the saltshaker on the table. There is the extra slice of chocolate cake on the plate. There is the cigarette in your hand.

The choices my patients make and the ways in which they approach their own health have shown me that an eighty-year-old recovering from heart surgery can sometimes be my healthiest patient, whereas a twenty-four-old on no medication can be my sickest. Wellness is partially about choice. Wellness is sometimes about change.

Wellness is a verb.

It was your idea in the first place.

So find your problem first.

And always look up.

Acknowledgments

This journey started with my colleagues at the Providence Heart and Vascular Institute at Providence St. Vincent Medical Center in Portland, Oregon. I am so proud to come to work every day with such an inspiring group of health care providers. You have supported my career and this venture from the very start. Ultimately, this book was written to benefit every person who walks through our doors.

Over two years ago, I began the process of putting my thoughts onto paper, and my brother recommended that I speak with our close friend Jonathan Zittrain, who has written several books. Jonathan was generous enough to put me in touch with Ike Williams at Kneerim & Williams Literary Agency, who would later become my agent. Jonathan has been so supportive of me during the past thirty years—thank you so much.

Ike and Editorial Manager Katherine Flynn were patient, supportive, and educational in helping me prepare my manuscript for submission, and I am so appreciative for their critical role in bringing this project from my desktop to the "real world" for consideration. Thank you for putting your trust in me.

And then Zachary Schisgal at Simon & Schuster made this opportunity a reality. Zach provided support and pushed me forward throughout every stage of edits and production. Zach truly gave me a chance, and I am forever grateful for his support and his friendship.

Jon Duke and Chuck Fox are two of the most amazing friends a person could hope for. Jon and I are constant dreamers, and I feel so lucky to share his energy. This project has made us closer as we thrive from each other's inspiration and new experiences. Chuck makes dreams reality every day—he is a dedicated, supportive, and selfless friend to me. You guys helped me so much.

I have met many new friends this year, from my colleagues at

WebMD.com, MedHelp.org, and Lifescript.com to people I have grown to know on Facebook and Twitter. In a world of e-mail, URL shorteners, and a growing landscape for making connections, I am amazed at the quality of people who I have met in these forums. I do not take these relationships for granted, and appreciate you all.

I am lucky that the most important relationships in my life are with my family. My parents Alan and Natalie are the most supportive, loving, and wonderful role models—they have made everything possible for me. I only hope that I do the same for my own boys. My brother, Jon, continues to be my greatest hero. There is nothing like having your big brother tell you he is proud of you. He is my best friend.

My beautiful sons Jack and Henry have truly made my life complete. They keep me grounded, inspired, and awestruck with every moment. I treasure them more than they will ever know. I want them to realize when they someday read this that they can accomplish anything, but the road itself proves to be a very satisfying goal.

Stacie, you are my life partner and holy grail. You are so patient, so understanding, so supportive, and so beautiful. I simply could not have done this or pretty much anything else without you in my corner. I love you.

The Solutions

TODAY

1. Commit yourself by taking a photo.
2. Join a support group.
3. Use automated reminders.
4. Tatango!
5. Get a commitment from your significant other.
6. Find a weight-loss buddy.
7. Follow people who inspire you on Twitter.
8. Become someone's coach.
9. Blog.
10. Call your doctor.
11. Weigh yourself daily.
12. Warm up.
13. Keep a food diary.
14. Drink six glasses of water a day.
15. Take a multivitamin.
16. Get your calcium.
17. Consider taking fish oil.
18. Look into probiotics.
19. Try taking whey protein after exercise.
20. Wear a pedometer.
21. Don't use exercise as a punishment.
22. Almonds.
23. Apples.
24. Grapes.
25. Greek yogurt.
26. Flaxseeds.
27. Pine nuts.

28. Enjoy 100-calorie snacks.
29. Don't overdose on energy bars.
30. Close the kitchen after dinner.
31. Sleep at least seven hours a night.

EVERY DAY

Eat

32. Eat breakfast every day.
33. Eat eggs twice a week.
34. Avoid bagels.
35. Eat healthier bread.
36. Switch to a healthier breakfast cereal.
37. Use spreads sparingly.
38. Scoop or go halfsies.
39. Limit your menu.
40. Don't eat out of vending machines.
41. Hold the mayonnaise.
42. Substitute a vegetable for French fries.
43. Don't eat and drive.
44. Use microwave meals.
45. Limit eating out to two days a week.
46. Don't eat while watching television.
47. Eat at the table.
48. Eat a salad most days of the week.
49. Start with soup at least twice a week.
50. Eat fish at least once a week.
51. Eat tofu once a week.
52. Eat leaner red meat.
53. Do chicken right.
54. Eat beans at least once a week.
55. Limit carbohydrate servings to one cup.
56. Limit takeout or delivery to once a week.

57. Store the leftovers first.
58. Serve meals restaurant style, not family style.
59. Serve meals as courses.
60. Make vegetables your main course.
61. Sneak vegetables into other foods.
62. Don't eat your children's food.
63. Use less salad dressing.
64. Put out a vegetable platter.
65. Unload your baked potato.
66. Cut the fat.
67. Substitute quinoa for rice.

Drink

68. Cut out sugar-sweetened beverages.
69. Avoid energy drinks.
70. Save your Starbucks.
71. Switch to skim.
72. Skip the diet soda.
73. Don't drink fruit juice.
74. Drink green tea.
75. Limit alcohol to weekends.

Exercise

76. Move slowly.
77. Push-ups.
78. The Hands Push.
79. The Fly.
80. Good Mornings.
81. The Bent-over Row.
82. Lateral Raises.
83. Chair dips.
84. Chair extensions.
85. Curls.
86. Squats.

87. Split squats.
88. Calf raises.
89. Standing twists.
90. The Tibetan Twist.
91. The Superman/Banana.

Act

92. Climb stairs for ten minutes each weekday.
93. Walk during breaks at work.
94. Walk after dinner.
95. Walk your dog every day.
96. Walk before you shop.

Live

97. Make grocery shopping a healthier exercise.
98. Outsmart the supermarket.
99. Buy canned fruits and vegetables without additional ingredients.
100. Read food labels.
101. Don't eat from the restaurant breadbasket.
102. Ask questions in restaurants.
103. When you buy in bulk, store in servings.
104. Avoid all-you-can-eat restaurants.
105. Give drive-throughs the drive-by.
106. Share an entrée when you go out to eat.
107. Avoid MSG.
108. Make your Mexican food healthier.
109. Ask for a doggy bag when you order your meal.
110. Order a better pizza.
111. Think outside the bun.
112. Go grocery shopping without your kids.

YOUR WAY

Eat

113. Fast.
114. Eat slowly.
115. Substitute lower-calorie and lower-fat cheese for what you are already buying.
116. Eat at least 25 grams of fiber each day.
117. Eat more protein at breakfast.
118. Add some spice.
119. Substitute fruit for cooking oil.
120. Ask for your sandwiches without cheese.
121. Use cooking spray.
122. Substitute for sour cream.
123. Stop using margarine and butter in cooking or as spreads.
124. Order smaller serving sizes.
125. *Hari hachi bu* one meal a day.
126. Clean out your freezer.
127. Know your serving size and eat one less.
128. Avoid white starches.
129. Order the children's meal at fast-food restaurants.
130. Consume less than 2,400 milligrams of sodium a day.
131. Eat your grapefruit.
132. Avoid anything with high-fructose corn syrup.
133. Eat rhubarb.
134. Don't use cheese as a garnish.
135. Skim oil and starch off the top when cooking.
136. Eat your largest meal of the day from a smaller plate.
137. Use bowls for snacks.
138. Pack your spouse's lunch.
139. Shop at a farmers' market once a week.
140. Splurge once a week on anything you like.

Drink

141. Don't use nondairy creamer.
142. Add ice.
143. Order wine by the glass.
144. Drink light beer.
145. Drink coffee instead of cocoa.
146. Drink additional water before going out to eat.
147. Cut out sugar substitutes.

Exercise

148. Move your exercise to the early morning.
149. Bicycle.
150. Join a sports league.
151. Run every other day.
152. Exercise during commercials.
153. Swim.
154. Add interval training to your workout.
155. Take up yoga.
156. Increase your time exercising by just one minute each week, and exercise faster.
157. Practice tai chi.
158. Race.
159. Dance.
160. Run barefoot.

Act

161. Get up, Get NEAT.
162. Take care of your own lawn.
163. Use trekking or walking poles.
164. Use hand weights while you walk.

Live

165. Meditate.
166. Use a financial incentive to reward your weight loss.

167. Play active video games.
168. Stop smoking marijuana.
169. Try acupuncture.
170. Change your commute.
171. Get hypnotized.
172. Chew gum four times a day.
173. Just watch the movie.
174. Change your environment to avoid temptation.
175. Reduce the amount of time you spend watching television.
176. Laugh for thirty minutes a day.
177. Wait twenty minutes before eating snacks or eating dessert.
178. Use blue.
179. Brighten your environment.
180. Listen to music while you exercise.
181. Brush your teeth after meals.
182. Turn off the Food Channel.
183. Buy a headset.
184. Say no to samples.
185. Bring your own airplane snacks.
186. Set the alarm on your computer.
187. Give your seat to someone else.
188. Kiss your partner ten times a day.
189. Don't order room service.
190. There's an app for that.
191. Clean out your closet.
192. Start a garden.
193. Make social outings active rather than food oriented.
194. Lobby to get menu calorie labeling in your area.
195. Use chopsticks.
196. Photograph your food.
197. Those shoes are made for walking.
198. See yourself thin.
199. Fill in the blank.
200. Count your blessings.

References

ABC News. "Poll: What Americans Eat for Breakfast"—May 17, 2005. www.abc news.go.com/gma/pollvault/story?id=762685.

Adams, K. F., et al. "Overweight, Obesity, and Mortality in a Large Prospective Cohort of Persons 50 to 71 Years Old." *New England Journal of Medicine* 355, no. 8 (2006): 763–78.

Andrade, A. M., et al. "Eating Slowly Led to Decreases in Energy Intake Within Meals in Healthy Women." *Journal of the American Dietetic Association* 108, no. 7 (2008): 1186–1191.

Auvichayapat, P., et al. "Effectiveness of Green Tea on Weight Reduction in Obese Thais: A Randomized, Controlled Trial." *Physiology & Behavior* 93, no. 3 (2008): 486–491.

Bailey, B., et al. "Energy Cost of ExerGaming in Adolescents." Paper presented at the annual meeting of the Obesity Society, October 3–7, 2008, Phoenix, AZ.

Baker, R. C., et al. "Weight Control During the Holidays: Highly Consistent Self-Monitoring as a Potentially Useful Coping Mechanism." *Health Psychology* 17, no. 4 (1998): 367–370.

Bassett, D. R., et al. "Energy Cost of Stair Climbing and Descending on the College Alumnus Questionnaire." *Medicine & Science in Sports & Exercise* 29, no. 9 (1997): 1250–1254.

Bassett, D. R., Jr. et al. "Walking, Cycling, and Obesity Rates in Europe, North America, and Australia." *Journal of Physical Activity and Health* 5, no. 6 (2008): 795–814.

Beers, E. A., et al. "Increasing Passive Energy Expenditure During Clerical Work." *European Journal of Applied Physiology* 103, no. 3 (2008): 353–360.

Beglinger, C., et al. "Fat in the Intestine as a Regulator of Appetite—Role of CCK." *Physiology & Behavior* 83, no. 4 (2004): 617–621.

Bellissimo, N., et al. "Effect of Television Viewing at Mealtime on Food Intake After a Glucose Preload in Boys." *Pediatric Research* 61, no. 6 (2007): 745–749.

Berg, C., et al. "Eating Patterns and Portion Size Associated with Obesity in a Swedish Population." *Appetite* 52, no. 1 (2009): 21–26.

Blanck, H. M., et al. "Factors Influencing Lunchtime Food Choices Among Working Americans." *Health Education & Behavior* 36, no. 2 (2009): 289–301.

Blass, E. M., et al. "On the Road to Obesity: Television Viewing Increases Intake of High-Density Foods." *Physiology & Behavior* 88, nos. 4–5 (2006): 597–604.

Bleich, S. N., et al. "Increasing Consumption of Sugar-Sweetened Beverages Among US Adults: 1988–1994 to 1999–2004." *American Journal of Clinical Nutrition* 89, no. 1 (2009): 372–381.

Boschmann, M., et al. "Water-Induced Thermogenesis." *Journal of Clinical Endocrinology & Metabolism* 88, no. 12 (2003): 6015–6019.

Boschmann, M., et al. "Water Drinking Induces Thermogenesis Through Osmosensitive Mechanisms." *Journal of Clinical Endocrinology & Metabolism* 92, no. 8 (2007): 3334–3337.

Braun, D. L., et al. "Bright Light Therapy Decreases Winter Binge Frequency in Women with Bulimia Nervosa: A Double-Blind, Placebo-Controlled Study." *Comprehensive Psychiatry* 40, no. 6 (1999): 442–448.

Bravata, D. M., et al. "Using Pedometers to Increase Physical Activity and Improve Health: A Systematic Review." *JAMA* 298, no. 19 (2007): 2296–2304.

Buchowski, M. S., et al. "Energy Expenditure of Genuine Laughter." *International Journal of Obesity* 31, no. 1 (2007): 131–137.

Burger, K. S., et al. "Characteristics of Self-Selected Portion Size in Young Adults." *Journal of the American Dietetic Association* 107, no. 4 (2007): 611–618.

Buscemi, D., et al. "Short Sleep Times Predict Obesity in Internal Medicine Clinic Patients." *Journal of Clinical Sleep Medicine* 3, no. 7 (2007): 681–688.

Butryn, M. L., et al. "Consistent Self-Monitoring of Weight: A Key Component of Successful Weight Loss Maintenance." *Obesity* 15, no. 12 (2007): 3091–3096.

Cabyoglu, M. T., et al. "The Treatment of Obesity by Acupuncture." *International Journal of Neuroscience* 116, no. 2 (2006): 165–175.

Campbell, W. W., et al. "Increased Energy Requirements and Changes in Body Composition with Resistance Training in Older Adults." *American Journal of Clinical Nutrition* 60, no. 2 (1994): 167–175.

Cappuccio, F. P., et al. "Meta-analysis of Short Sleep Duration and Obesity in Children and Adults." *Sleep* 31, no. 5 (2008): 619–626.

Cepoiu, M., et al. "Recognition of Depression by Non-psychiatric Physicians—a Systematic Literature Review and Meta-analysis." *Journal of General Internal Medicine* 23, no. 1 (2008): 25–36.

Chavis, S. "I'm a 225-Pound Weight-Loss Editor. Get Over It." http://diet .com/2009/01/08/im-a-225-pound-weight-loss-editor-get-over-it.

Cleland, V. J., et al. "Television Viewing and Abdominal Obesity in Young Adults: Is the Association Mediated by Food and Beverage Consumption During Viewing Time or Reduced Leisure-Time Physical Activity?" *American Journal of Clinical Nutrition* 87, no. 5 (2008): 1148–1155.

Creaton, H., ed. *Victorian Diaries: The Daily Lives of Victorian Men and Women.* London: Mitchell Beazley, 2001.

Cummings, D. E., et al. "Plasma Ghrelin Levels After Diet-Induced Weight Loss or Gastric Bypass Surgery." *New England Journal of Medicine* 346, no. 21 (2002): 1623–1630.

de Oliveira, M. C., et al. "A Low-Energy-Dense Diet Adding Fruit Reduces Weight and Energy Intake in Women." *Appetite* 51, no. 2 (2008): 291–295.

de Oliveira, M. C., et al. "Weight Loss Associated with a Daily Intake of Three Apples or Three Pears Among Overweight Women." *Nutrition* 19, no. 3 (2003): 253–256.

Dechamps, A., et al. "Pilot Study of a 10-Week Multidisciplinary Tai Chi Intervention in Sedentary Obese Women." *Clinical Journal of Sport Medicine* 19, no. 1 (2009): 49–53.

Deibert, P., et al. "Weight Loss Without Losing Muscle Mass in Pre-obese and Obese Subjects Induced by a High-Soy-Protein Diet." *International Journal of Obesity and Related Metabolic Disorders* 28, no. 10 (2004): 1349–1352.

Diliberti, N., et al. "Increased Portion Size Leads to Increased Energy Intake in a Restaurant Meal." *Obesity Research* 12, no. 3 (2004): 562–568.

Driskell, J. A., et al. "Using Nutrition Labeling as a Potential Tool for Changing Eating Habits of University Dining Hall Patrons. *Journal of the American Dietary Association* 108, no. 12 (2008): 2071–2076.

Dulloo, A. G., et al. "Normal Caffeine Consumption: Influence on Thermogenesis and Daily Energy Expenditure in Lean and Postobese Human Volunteers." *American Journal of Clinical Nutrition* 49, no. 1 (1989): 44–50.

Dunai, A., et al. "Moderate Exercise and Bright Light Treatment in Overweight and Obese Individuals." *Obesity* 15, no. 7 (2007): 1749–1757.

Ebbeling, C. B., et al. "Effects of Decreasing Sugar-Sweetened Beverage Consumption on Body Weight in Adolescents: A Randomized, Controlled Pilot Study." *Pediatrics* 117, no. 3 (2006): 673–680.

Emmons, Robert A. *Thanks! How the New Science of Gratitude Can Make You Happier.* Boston: Houghton Mifflin, 2007.

Epstein, L. H., et al. "A Randomized Trial of the Effects of Reducing Television Viewing and Computer Use on Body Mass Index in Young Children." *Archives of Pediatric and Adolescent Medicine* 162, no. 3 (2008): 239–245.

Finkelstein, E. A., et al. "A Pilot Study Testing the Effect of Different Levels of Financial Incentives on Weight Loss Among Overweight Employees." *Journal of Occupational and Environmental Medicine* 49, no. 9 (2007): 981–989.

Flood, J. E., et al. "Soup Preloads in a Variety of Forms Reduce Meal Energy Intake." *Appetite* 49, no. 3 (2007): 626–634.

Foltin, R. W., et al. "Behavioral Analysis of Marijuana Effects on Food Intake in Humans." *Pharmacology Biochemistry and Behavior* 25, no. 3 (1986): 577–582.

Foltin, R. W., et al. "Effects of Smoked Marijuana on Food Intake and Body Weight of Humans Living in a Residential Laboratory." *Appetite* 11, no. 1 (1988): 1–14.

Fowler, S. P., et al. "Fueling the Obesity Epidemic? Artificially Sweetened Beverage Use and Long-Term Weight Gain." *Obesity* 16, no. 8 (2008): 1894–1900.

Fraser, G. E., et al. "Effect on Body Weight of a Free 76 Kilojoule (320 Calorie) Daily Supplement of Almonds for Six Months." *Journal of the American College of Nutrition* 21, no. 3 (2002): 275–283.

Frestedt, J. L., et al. "A Whey-Protein Supplement Increases Fat Loss and Spares Lean Muscle in Obese Subjects: A Randomized Human Clinical Study." *Nutrition & Metabolism* 5, no. 8 (2008): 5–8.

Fujioka, K., et al. "The Effects of Grapefruit on Weight and Insulin Resistance: Relationship to the Metabolic Syndrome." *Journal of Medicinal Food* 9, no. 1 (2006): 49–54.

Gaesser, G. A. "Carbohydrate Quantity and Quality in Relation to Body Mass Index." *Journal of the American Dietetic Association* 107, no. 10 (2007): 1768–1780.

Gappmaier, E., et al. "Aerobic Exercise in Water Versus Walking on Land: Effects on Indices of Fat Reduction and Weight Loss of Obese Women." *Journal of Sports Medicine and Physical Fitness* 46, no. 4 (2006): 564–569.

Goldstein, D. J., et al. "Fluoxetine: A Randomized Clinical Trial in the Treatment of Obesity." *International Journal of Obesity and Related Metabolic Disorders* 18, no. 3 (1994): 129–135.

Gorin, A. A., et al. "Home Grocery Delivery Improves the Household Food Environments of Behavioral Weight Loss Participants: Results of an 8-Week Pilot Study." *International Journal of Behavioral Nutrition and Physical Activity* 4, no. 58 (2007).

Gorin, A. A., et al. "Involving Support Partners in Obesity Treatment." *Journal of Consulting and Clinical Psychology* 73, no. 2 (2005): 341–343.

Gorin, A. A., et al. "Weight Loss Treatment Influences Untreated Spouses and the Home Environment: Evidence of a Ripple Effect." *International Journal of Obesity* 32, no. 11 (2008): 1678–1684.

Greenberg, I., et al. "Effects of Marihuana Use on Body Weight and Caloric Intake in Humans." *Psychopharmacology* (Berlin) 49, no. 1 (1976): 79–84.

Gregory, S. "Fast Food: Would You Like 1,000 Calories with That?" June 29, 2009. www.time.com.

Grimaldi, S., et al. "Experienced Poor Lighting Contributes to the Seasonal Fluctuations in Weight and Appetite That Relate to the Metabolic Syndrome." *Journal of Environmental and Public Health*, 2009, article ID 165013.

Hamer, M., et al. "Active Commuting and Cardiovascular Risk: A Meta-analytic Review." *Preventive Medicine* 46, no. 1 (2008): 9–13.

Hampton, T. "Sugar Substitutes Linked to Weight Gain." *JAMA* 299, no. 18 (2008): 2137–2138.

Hamwi, G. J. "Therapy: Changing Dietary Concepts." In *Diabetes Mellitus: Diagnosis and Treatment*, Vol. 1, edited by T. S. Danowski. New York: American Diabetes Association, 1964.

Hannum, S. M., et al. "Use of Packaged Entrees as Part of a Weight-Loss Diet in Overweight Men: An 8-week Randomized Clinical Trial." *Diabetes, Obesity and Metabolism* 8, no. 2 (2006): 146–155.

Harris, J. L., et al. "Priming Effects of Television Food Advertising on Eating Behavior." *Health Psychology* 28, no. 4 (2009): 404–413.

He, K., et al. "Association of Monosodium Glutamate Intake with Overweight in Chinese Adults: The INTERMAP Study." *Obesity* 16, no. 8 (2008): 1875–1880.

Hetherington, M. M., et al. "Short-Term Effects of Chewing Gum on Snack Intake and Appetite." *Appetite* 48, no. 3 (2007): 397–401.

Hill, A. M., et al. "Combining Fish-Oil Supplements with Regular Aerobic Exercise Improves Body Composition and Cardiovascular Disease Risk Factors." *American Journal of Clinical Nutrition* 85, no. 5 (2007): 1267–1274.

Hollis, J. F., et al. "Weight Loss During the Intensive Intervention Phase of the Weight-Loss Maintenance Trial." *American Journal of Preventive Medicine* 35, no. 2 (2008): 118–126.

Holt, S. H., et al. "The Effects of Equal-Energy Portions of Different Breads on Blood Glucose Levels, Feelings of Fullness and Subsequent Food Intake." *Journal of the American Dietetic Association* 101, no. 7 (2001): 767–773.

Howarth, N. C., et al. "Dietary Fiber and Weight Regulation." *Nutrition Reviews* 59, no. 5 (2001): 129–139.

Hrovat, K. B., et al. "The New Food Label, Type of Fat, and Consumer Choice: A Pilot Study." *Archives of Family Medicine* 3, no. 8 (1994): 690–695.

Hsu, C. H., et al. "Electroacupuncture in Obese Women: A Randomized, Controlled Pilot Study." *Journal of Women's Health* 14, no. 5 (2005): 434–440.

Huang, T. T., et al. "Reading Nutrition Labels and Fat Consumption in Adolescents." *Journal of Adolescent Health* 35, no. 5 (2004): 399–401.

Hurling, R., et al. "Using Internet and Mobile Phone Technology to Deliver an Automated Physical Activity Program: Randomized Controlled Trial." *Journal of Medical Internet Research* 9, no. 2 (2007): e7.

Jason, L. A., et al. "A Large-Scale, Short-Term, Media-Based Weight Loss Program." *American Journal of Health Promotion* 5, no. 6 (1991): 432–437.

Jenkins, D., et al. "Dose Response of Almonds on Coronary Heart Disease Risk Factors: Blood Lipids, Oxidized Low-Density Lipoproteins, Lipoprotein(a), Homocysteine, and Pulmonary Nitric Oxide." *Circulation* 106 (2002): 1327–1332.

Johnson, N. P., et al. "Relation of Exercise Capacity and Body Mass Index to Mortality in Patients with Intermediate to High Risk of Coronary Artery Disease." *American Journal of Cardiology* 102, no. 8 (2008): 1028–1033.

Johnstone, A. M. "Fasting—the Ultimate Diet?" *Obesity Reviews* 8, no. 3 (2007): 211–222.

Joo, N., and B. Kim. "Mobile Phone Short Message Service Messaging for Behaviour Modification in a Community-Based Weight Control Programme in Korea." *Journal of Telemedicine and Telecare* 13, no. 8 (2007): 416–420.

Kant, A. K., et al. "Eating Out in America, 1987–2000: Trends and Nutritional Correlates." *Preventive Medicine* 38, no. 2 (2004): 243–249.

Kimmons, J. E., et al. "Multivitamin Use in Relation to Self-Reported Body Mass Index and Weight Loss Attempts." *MedGenMed* 8, no. 3 (2006): 3.

Kimmons, J. E., et al. "Associations Between Body Mass Index and the Prevalence of Low Micronutrient Levels Among US Adults." *MedGenMed* 8, no. 4 (2006): 59.

Kirsch, I. "Hypnotic Enhancement of Cognitive-Behavioral Weight Loss Treatment: Another Meta-reanalysis." *Journal of Consulting and Clinical Psychology* 64, no. 3 (1996): 517–519.

Kobriger, S. L., et al. "The Contribution of Golf to Daily Physical Activity Recommendations: How Many Steps Does It Take to Complete a Round of Golf?" *Mayo Clinic Proceedings* 81, no. 8 (2006): 1041–1043.

Koot, P., et al. "Comparison of Changes in Energy Expenditure and Body Temperatures After Caffeine Consumption." *Annals of Nutritional Metabolism* 39, no. 3 (1995): 135–142.

Kreuter, M. W., et al. "Do Nutrition Label Readers Eat Healthier Diets? Behavioral Correlates of Adults' Use of Food Labels." *American Journal of Preventive Medicine* 13, no. 4 (1997): 277–283.

Kristal, A. R., et al. "Predictors of Self-Initiated, Healthful Dietary Change." *Journal of the American Dietetic Association* 101, no. 7 (2001): 762–766.

Kristensen, M., et al. "Whole Flaxseeds but Not Sunflower Seeds in Rye Bread Reduce Apparent Digestibility of Fat in Healthy Volunteers." *European Journal of Clinical Nutrition* 62, no. 8 (2008): 961–967.

Kromhout, D., et al. "Physical Activity and Dietary Fiber Determine Population Body Fat Levels: The Seven Countries Study." *International Journal of Obesity and Related Metabolic Disorders* 25, no. 3 (2001): 301–306.

Kronenberg, F., et al. "Influence of Leisure Time Physical Activity and Television Watching on Atherosclerosis Risk Factors in the NHLBI Family Heart Study." *Atherosclerosis* 153, no. 2 (2000): 433–443.

Kuo, T., et al. "Menu Labeling as a Potential Strategy for Combating the Obesity Epidemic: A Health Impact Assessment." *American Journal of Public Health* 99, no. 9 (2009): 1680–1686.

Lam, R. W., et al. "A Controlled Study of Light Therapy for Bulimia Nervosa." *American Journal of Psychiatry* 151 (1994): 744–750.

Lanningham-Foster, L., et al. "Labor Saved, Calories Lost: The Energetic Impact of Domestic Labor-Saving Devices." *Obesity Research* 11, no. 10 (2003): 1178–1181.

Leidy, H. J., et al. "Circulating Ghrelin Is Sensitive to Changes in Body Weight During a Diet and Exercise Program in Normal-Weight Young Women." *Journal of Clinical Endocrinology & Metabolism* 89, no. 6 (2004): 2659–2664.

Levine, J., et al. "The Energy Expended in Chewing Gum." *New England Journal of Medicine* 342, no. 2 (2000): 1531.

Levine, J. A., et al. "Interindividual Variation in Posture Allocation: Possible Role in Human Obesity." *Science* 307, no. 5709 (2005): 584–586.

Levine, J. A., et al. "Non-Exercise Activity Thermogenesis: The Crouching Tiger Hidden Dragon of Societal Weight Gain." *Arteriosclerosis, Thrombosis, and Vascular Biology* 26, no. 4 (2006): 729–736.

Levitsky, D. A., et al. "Monitoring Weight Daily Blocks the Freshman Weight Gain: A Model for Combating the Epidemic of Obesity." *International Journal of Obesity* 30, no. 6 (2006): 1003–1010.

Liao, F. H., et al. "Effectiveness of a Soy-Based Compared with a Traditional Low-Calorie Diet on Weight Loss and Lipid Levels in Overweight Adults." *Nutrition* 23, nos. 7–8 (2007): 551–556.

Linde, J. A., et al. "Relation of Body Mass Index to Depression and Weighing Frequency in Overweight Women." *Preventive Medicine* 45, no. 1 (2007): 75–79.

Linde, J. A., et al. "Self-Weighing in Weight Gain Prevention and Weight Loss Trials." *Annals of Behavioral Medicine* 30, no. 3 (2005): 210–216.

Liu, S., et al. "Relation Between Changes in Intakes of Dietary Fiber and Grain Products and Changes in Weight and Development of Obesity Among Middle-Aged Women." *American Journal of Clinical Nutrition* 78, no. 5 (2003): 920–927.

Love, J. A., et al. "Nutrient Composition and Sensory Attributes of Cooked Ground Beef: Effects of Fat Content, Cooking Method, and Water Rinsing." *Journal of the American Dietetic Association* 92, no. 11 (1992): 1367–1371.

Ludwig, D. S., et al. "Dietary Fiber, Weight Gain, and Cardiovascular Disease Risk Factors in Young Adults." *JAMA*, 282, no. 16 (1999): 1539–1546.

Lyons, E., et al. "Energy Expenditure During Wii Sports Minigames in Overweight Children: Comparing Data Parameter Selection." Paper presented at the annual meeting of the Obesity Society, October 3–7, 2008, Phoenix, AZ.

Maddison, R., et al. "Energy Expended Playing Video Console Games: An Opportunity to Increase Children's Physical Activity?" *Pediatric Exercise Science* 19, no. 3 (2007): 334–343.

Magee, E. "The Best Bread: Tips for Buying Breads." www.webmd.com/food.

———. "Choosing a Healthy Breakfast Cereal." www.webmd.com/food.

Mahajan, A. S., et al. "Lipid Profile of Coronary Risk Subjects Following Yogic Lifestyle Intervention." *Indian Heart Journal* 51 (1999): 37–40.

Maki, K. C., et al. "Green Tea Catechin Consumption Enhances Exercise-Induced Abdominal Fat Loss in Overweight and Obese Adults." *Journal of Nutrition* 139, no. 2 (2009): 264–270.

Major, G. C., et al. "Calcium Plus Vitamin D Supplementation and Fat Mass Loss in Female Very Low-Calcium Consumers: Potential Link with a Calcium-Specific Appetite Control." *British Journal of Nutrition* 101, no. 5 (2009): 659–663.

Major, G. C., et al. "Multivitamin and Dietary Supplements, Body Weight and Appetite: Results from a Cross-sectional and a Randomized Double-Blind Placebo-Controlled Study." *British Journal of Nutrition* 99, no. 5 (2008): 1157–1167.

Malik, V. S., et al. "Intake of Sugar-Sweetened Beverages and Weight Gain: A Systematic Review." *American Journal of Clinical Nutrition* 84, no. 2 (2006): 274–288.

Manchanda S. C., et al. "Retardation of Coronary Atherosclerosis with Yoga Lifestyle Intervention. *Journal of the Association of Physicians in India* 48, no. 7: 687–694.

Marmonier, C., et al. "Snacks Consumed in a Nonhungry State Have Poor Satiating Efficiency: Influence of Snack Composition on Substrate Utilization and Hunger." *American Journal of Clinical Nutrition* 76, no. 3 (2002): 518–528.

Martin, C. K., et al. "Slower Eating Rate Reduces the Food Intake of Men, but Not Women: Implications for Behavioral Weight Control." *Behavioral Research and Therapy* 45, no. 10 (2007): 2349–2359.

Maruyama, K., et al. "The Joint Impact on Being Overweight of Self Reported Behaviours of Eating Quickly and Eating Until Full: Cross Sectional Survey." *BMJ* 2008; 337: a2002.

Meyer, A. M., et al. "Television, Physical Activity, Diet, and Body Weight Status: The ARIC Cohort." *International Journal of Behavioral Nutrition and Physical Activity* 5 (2008): 68.

Micco, N., et al. "Minimal In-person Support as an Adjunct to Internet Obesity Treatment." *Annals of Behavioral Medicine* 33, no. 1 (2007): 49–56.

Miyatake, N., et al. "Daily Walking Reduces Visceral Adipose Tissue Areas and Improves Insulin Resistance in Japanese Obese Subjects." *Diabetes Research and Clinical Practice* 58, no. 2 (2002): 101–107.

Mourao, D. M., et al. "Effects of Food Form on Appetite and Energy Intake in Lean and Obese Young Adults." *International Journal of Obesity* 31, no. 11 (2007): 1688–1695.

Murphy, J. M., et al. "Obesity and Weight Gain in Relation to Depression: Findings from the Stirling County Study." *International Journal of Obesity* 33, no. 3 (2009): 335–341.

Myers, J., et al. "Exercise Capacity and Mortality Among Men Referred for Exercise Testing." *New England Journal of Medicine* 346, no. 11 (2002): 793–801.

Nagao, T., et al. "A Green Tea Extract High in Catechins Reduces Body Fat and Cardiovascular Risks in Humans." *Obesity* 15, no. 6 (2007): 1473–1483.

Nagao, T., et al. "Ingestion of a Tea Rich in Catechins Leads to a Reduction in Body Fat and Malondialdehyde-Modified LDL in Men." *American Journal of Clinical Nutrition* 81, no. 1 (2005): 122–129.

Nettleton, J. A., et al. "Diet Soda Intake and Risk of Incident Metabolic Syndrome and Type 2 Diabetes in the Multi-Ethnic Study of Atherosclerosis." *Diabetes Care* 32, no. 4 (2009): 688–694.

Nielsen, S. J., and B. M. Popkin. "Changes in Beverage Intake Between 1977 and 2001." *American Journal of Preventive Medicine* 27, no. 3 (2004): 205–210.

Nielsen, S. J., et al. "Patterns and Trends in Food Portion Sizes, 1977–1998." *JAMA* 289, no. 4 (2003): 450–453.

Nguyen, T. T., et al. "Cholesterol-Lowering Effect of Stanol Ester in a US Population of Mildly Hypercholesterolemic Men and Women: A Randomized Controlled Trial." *Mayo Clinic Proceedings* 74, no. 12 (1999): 1198–1206.

NPD Group. Survey of 3,500 respondents to the question "What did I order at a restaurant today?" as part of a year-long diary of eating habits in 2004. www.usatoday.com/money/industries/food/2005-05-12-bad-food-cover_x.htm.

Oberlinner, C., et al. "Prevention of Overweight and Obesity in the Workplace. BASF Health Promotion Campaign 'Trim Down the Pounds—Losing Weight Without Losing Your Mind.'" *Gesundheitswesen* 69, no. 7 (2007): 385–392.

Ogden, C., et al. "Prevalence of Overweight and Obesity in the United States, 1999–2004." *JAMA* 295 (2006): 1549–1555.

Orth, W. S., et al. "Support Group Meeting Attendance Is Associated with Better Weight Loss." *Obesity Surgery* 18, no. 4 (2008): 391–394.

Ostmann, E., et al. "Vinegar Supplementation Lowers Glucose and Insulin Responses and Increases Satiety After a Bread Meal in Healthy Subjects." *European Journal of Clinical Nutrition* 59, no. 9 (2005): 983–988.

Otsuka, R., et al. "Eating Fast Leads to Obesity: Findings Based on Self-Administered Questionnaires Among Middle-Aged Japanese Men and Women." *Journal of Epidemiology* 16, no. 3 (2006): 117–124.

Palank, E. A., et al. "The Benefits of Walking the Golf Course: Effects on Lipoprotein Levels and Risk Ratios." *The Physician and Sportsmedicine* 18, no. 10 (1990): 77–80.

Parkkari, J., et al. "A Controlled Trial of the Health Benefits of Regular Walking on a Golf Course." *American Journal of Medicine* 109, no. 2 (2008): 102–108.

Pasman, W. J., et al. "The Effect of Korean Pine Nut Oil on In Vitro CCK Release, on Appetite Sensations and on Gut Hormones in Post-menopausal Overweight Women." *Lipids in Health and Disease* 7 (2008): 10.

Patrick, K., et al. "A Text Message–Based Intervention for Weight Loss: Randomized Controlled Trial." *Journal of Medical Internet Research* 11, no. 1 (2009): e1.

Paul-Ebhohimhen, V., and A. Avenell. "Systematic Review of the Use of Financial Incentives in Treatments for Obesity and Overweight." *Obesity Reviews* 9, no. 4 (2008): 355–367.

Porcari, J. P., et al. "The Physiological Responses to Walking with and without Power Poles on Treadmill Exercise." *Research Quarterly for Exercise & Sport* 68, no. 2 (1997): 161–166.

Richardson, C. R., et al. "A Meta-analysis of Pedometer-Based Walking Interventions and Weight Loss." *Annals of Family Medicine* 6, no. 1 (2008): 69–77.

Rodondi, N., et al. "Marijuana Use, Diet, Body Mass Index, and Cardiovascular Risk Factors (from the CARDIA Study)." *American Journal of Cardiology* 98, no. 4 (2006): 478–484.

Rolls, B. J., et al. "Provision of Foods Differing in Energy Density Affects Long-Term Weight Loss." *Obesity Research* 13, no. 6 (2005): 1052–1060.

Rolls, B. J., et al. "Salad and Satiety: Energy Density and Portion Size of a First-Course Salad Affect Energy Intake at Lunch." *Journal of the American Dietetic Association* 104, no. 10 (2004): 1570–1576.

Rozin, P., et al. "The Ecology of Eating: Smaller Portion Sizes in France Than in the United States Help Explain the French Paradox." *Psychological Science* 14, no. 5 (2003): 450–454.

Sacks, F. M., et al. "Comparison of Weight-Loss Diets with Different Compositions of Fat, Protein, and Carbohydrates." *New England Journal of Medicine* 360, no. 9 (2009): 859–873.

Sartorelli, D. S., et al. "High Intake of Fruits and Vegetables Predicts Weight Loss in Brazilian Overweight Adults." *Nutrition Research* 28, no. 4 (2008): 233–238.

Schlundt, D. G., et al. "The Role of Breakfast in the Treatment of Obesity: A Randomized Clinical Trial." *American Journal of Clinical Nutrition* 55, no. 3 (1992): 645–651.

Schmidt, T., et al. "Changes in Cardiovascular Risk Factors and Hormones During a Comprehensive Residential Three Month Kriya Yoga Training and Vegetarian Nutrition." *Acta Physiologica Scandinavica* 640 (1997): S158–S162.

Schneider, K. L., et al. "Design and Methods for a Randomized Clinical Trial Treating Comorbid Obesity and Major Depressive Disorder." *BMC Psychiatry* 8 (2008): 877.

Sheldahl, L. M., et al. "Responses of People with Coronary Artery Disease to Common Lawn-Care Tasks." *European Journal of Applied Physiology and Occupational Physiology* 72, no. 4 (1996): 357–364.

Shenassa, E. D., et al. "Routine Stair Climbing in Place of Residence and Body Mass Index: A Pan-European Population Based Study." *International Journal of Obesity* 32, no. 3 (2008): 490–494.

Shephard, R. J. "Is Active Commuting the Answer to Population Health?" *Sports Medicine* 38, no. 9 (2008): 751–758.

Shimamoto, H., et al. "Low Impact Aerobic Dance as a Useful Exercise Mode for Reducing Body Mass in Mildly Obese Middle-Aged Women." *Applied Human Science* 17, no. 3 (1998): 109–114.

Shiraishi, T., et al. "Effects of Bilateral Auricular Acupuncture Stimulation on Body Weight in Healthy Volunteers and Mildly Obese Patients." *Experimental Biology and Medicine* 228, no. 10 (2003): 1201–1207.

Singh, M., et al. "The Association Between Obesity and Short Sleep Duration: A Population-Based Study." *Journal of Clinical Sleep Medicine* 1, no. 4 (2005): 357–363.

Stookey, J. D., et al. "Drinking Water Is Associated with Weight Loss in Overweight Dieting Women Independent of Diet and Activity." *Obesity* 16, no. 11 (2008): 2481–2488.

Stradling, J., et al. "Controlled Trial of Hypnotherapy for Weight Loss in Patients with Obstructive Sleep Apnoea." *International Journal of Obesity Related Metabolic Disorders* 22, no. 3 (1988): 278–281.

Stroebele, N., et al. "Do 100 Calorie Snack Packs Help Control Snacking Behavior?" Paper presented at the annual meeting of the Obesity Society, October 3–7, 2008, Phoenix, AZ.

Swithers, S. E., et al. "A Role for Sweet Taste: Calorie Predictive Relations in Energy Regulation by Rats." *Behavioral Neuroscience* 122, no. 1 (2008): 161–173.

Taheri, S., et al. "Short Sleep Duration Is Associated with Reduced Leptin, Elevated Ghrelin, and Increased Body Mass Index." *PLoS Medicine* 1, no. 3 (2004): e62.

Tanco, S., et al. "Well-being and Morbid Obesity in Women: A Controlled Therapy Evaluation." *International Journal of Eating Disorders* 23, no. 3 (1998): 325–339.

Teh, K. C., et al. "Heart Rate, Oxygen Uptake, and Energy Cost of Ascending and Descending the Stairs." *Medicine of Science in Sports & Exercise* 34, no. 4 (2002): 695–699.

Thorsdottir, I., et al. "Randomized Trial of Weight-Loss Diets for Young Adults Varying in Fish and Fish Oil Content." *International Journal of Obesity* 31, no. 10 (2007): 1560–1566.

U.S. Centers for Disease Control and Prevention, National Center for Health Statistics. *Health, United States, 2006.* (prepublication). www.cdc.gov/nchs/hus.htm.

U.S. Department of Health and Human Services. "The Surgeon General's Call to Action to Prevent and Decrease Overweight and Obesity: Overweight in Children and Adolescents." www.surgeongeneral.gov/topics/obesity/calltoaction/fact_adolescents.htm.

U.S. National Institutes of Health, National Institute of Diabetes and Digestive and Kidney Diseases. "Statistics Related to Overweight and Obesity: Economic Costs." February 2010. http://win.niddk.nih.gov/statistics/index.htm.

Vander Wal, J. S., et al. "Egg Breakfast Enhances Weight Loss." *International Journal of Obesity* 32, no. 10 (2008): 1545–1551.

Vander Wal, J. S., et al. "Short-Term Effect of Eggs on Satiety in Overweight and Obese Subjects." *Journal of the American College of Nutrition* 24, no. 6 (2005): 510–515.

Volpp, K. G., et al. "Financial Incentive-Based Approaches for Weight Loss: A Randomized Trial." *JAMA* 300, no. 22 (2008): 2631–2637.

Walter, P. R., et al. "Acute Responses to Using Walking Poles in Patients with Coronary Artery Disease." *Journal of Cardiopulmonary Rehabilitation* 16, no. 4 (1996): 245–250.

Wansink, B., et al. "Bad Popcorn in Big Buckets: Portion Size Can Influence Intake as Much as Taste." *Journal of Nutrition Education and Behavior* 37, no. 5 (2005): 242–245.

Wansink, B., et al. "Bottomless Bowls: Why Visual Cues of Portion Size May Influence Intake." *Obesity Research* 13, no. 1 (2005): 93–100.

Wansink, B., et al. "Eating Behavior and Obesity at Chinese Buffets." *Obesity* 16, no. 8 (2008): 1957–1960.

Wansink, B., et al. "Ice Cream Illusions: Bowls, Spoons, and Self-Served Portion Sizes." *American Journal of Preventive Medicine* 31, no. 3 (2006): 240–243.

Wansink, B., et al. "The Office Candy Dish: Proximity's Influence on Estimated and Actual Consumption." *International Journal of Obesity* 30, no. 5 (2006): 871–875.

Wansink, B., et al. "Super Bowls: Serving Bowl Size and Food Consumption." *JAMA* 293, no. 14 (2005): 1727–1728.

Wardle, J., et al. "Nutrition Knowledge and Food Intake." *Appetite* 34, no. 3 (2000): 269–275.

Wells, H. F., and J. Busby. "Americans' Dairy Consumption Below Recommendations." *Amber Waves,* November 2007.

White, E., et al. "Dietary Changes Among Husbands of Participants in a Low-Fat Dietary Intervention." *American Journal of Preventive Medicine* 7, no. 5 (1991): 319–325.

Wien, M. A., et al. "Almonds vs. Complex Carbohydrates in a Weight Reduction Program." *International Journal of Obesity and Related Metabolic Disorders* 27, no. 11 (2003): 1365–1372.

World Health Organization. "Controlling the Global Obesity Epidemic." http://www.who.int/nutrition/topics/obesity/en/index.html.

Zemel, M. B., et al. "Dairy Augmentation of Total and Central Fat Loss in Obese Subjects." *International Journal of Obesity* 29, no. 4 (2005): 391–397.

Zemel, M. B., et al. "Effects of Calcium and Dairy on Body Composition and Weight Loss in African-American Adults." *Obesity Research* 13, no. 7 (2005): 1218–1225.

Zepeda, L. "Think Before You Eat: Photographic Food Diaries as Intervention Tools to Change Dietary Decision Making and Attitudes." *International Journal of Consumer Studies* 32, no. 6 (2008): 692–698.

Index